BEYOND HOT YOGA

BEYOND HOT YOGA

ON PATTERNS, PRACTICE, AND MOVEMENT

WITH AN ILLUSTRATED GUIDE TO A NEW RITUALIZED YOGA SEQUENCE

KYLE FERGUSON
WITH ANTHONY GRUDIN

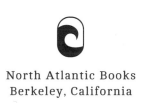

North Atlantic Books
Berkeley, California

Published by
North Atlantic Books
Berkeley, California

Cover design by Jess Morphew
Interior photos by Andy Duback
Book design by Happenstance Type-O-Rama

Printed in the United States of America

Beyond Hot Yoga: On Patterns, Practice, and Movement is sponsored and published by North Atlantic Books, an educational nonprofit based in Berkeley, California, that collaborates with partners to develop cross-cultural perspectives, nurture holistic views of art, science, the humanities, and healing, and seed personal and global transformation by publishing work on the relationship of body, spirit, and nature.

North Atlantic Books' publications are distributed to the US trade and internationally by Penguin Random House Publishers Services. For further information, visit our website at www.northatlanticbooks.com.

Library of Congress Cataloging-in-Publication Data

Names: Ferguson, Kyle, 1983– author. | Grudin, Anthony, 1976– author.
Title: Beyond hot yoga : on patterns, practice, and movement : with an
    illustrated guide to a new ritualized yoga sequence / Kyle Ferguson with
    Anthony Grudin.
Description: Berkeley, California : North Atlantic Books, 2021. | Summary:
    "A holistic method for practicing hot yoga that offers a new series of
    postures based on a modern understanding of anatomy and movement"—
    Provided by publisher.
Identifiers: LCCN 2020045811 (print) | LCCN 2020045812 (ebook) | ISBN
    9781623175948 (paperback) | ISBN 9781623175955 (epub)
Subjects: LCSH: Hatha yoga. | Thermotherapy.
Classification: LCC RA781.7 .F47 2021 (print) | LCC RA781.7 (ebook) | DDC
    613.7/046—dc23
LC record available at https://lccn.loc.gov/2020045811
LC ebook record available at https://lccn.loc.gov/2020045812

1 2 3 4 5 6 7 8 9 KPC 26 25 24 23 22 21

For the Second Circle Yoga family

CONTENTS

PART 2: PRACTICE: THE FOUNDATIONS OF REPATTERNING (A.K.A. "FOUNDATIONS")

PART 3: A THEORY OF RELATIVITY IN THE TIME OF EXPONENTIAL GROWTH

APPENDIX

ACKNOWLEDGMENTS

From Kyle

Please don't hold any of these against anyone. They tried their best.

First, I want to thank my parents. Mom and Dad, thank you for letting me be weird, for holding out faith, and for always finding the high ground. You made some intense kids with crazy brains. I'm humbled by your patience, commitment, and love.

To my siblings, you make this ride rich and true. Katey, thank you for being my anchor person. I have needed it often and you've never faltered. Schuyler, thank you for inspiring me to look at the world differently. You have always pushed me to be better, and it almost worked that one time. Jack, you're the worst. I cannot abide your capacity to actually make sacrifices—life-size sacrifices—for others. If you weren't my role model, I would be really mad at you right now.

To my cowriter Anthony, thank you for getting me to do this. This here book would never have existed without your constant encouragement and steady hand. It has been a wild ride from hastily composed proposals to conceptual overhauls, to sea changes in the mission, to new titles, to print. You have been a careful shepherd to the clamorous flock of rabid emus that is my mind.

Likewise, thank you to Gillian and Alison at North Atlantic for believing in this project and guiding it through all of its forms.

To the Second Circle Yoga family of students, teachers, and founders; thank you for getting aboard this steamboat, giving it ballast and fuel, and riding it with me straight into the wall. To my co-teachers, Betsy,

Emily, Robert, and Summer, you are remarkable, intelligent leaders and steadfast friends. You ended up teaching me in the end, and what I got was way more valuable. I love you all.

To all of my teachers, I'm forever grateful. My sincere apologies if I missed the actual point; I have that problem sometimes. Also, thanks to Noah Gabriel-Landis at Priority Strength (http://prioritystrength.com) for help reviewing the material. And a special thanks to our amazing photo models, Robert, Betsy, Summer, Emily, Isaiah, Marnie, Chris, Rachael, Bo, and Sarah.

To my friends, hi! Thank you for showing me what it looks like to be good in the world. You'd better read my book or we are super broken up. Also, come do yoga.

Finally, to all of the students I have worked with throughout the years; thank you for practicing. You are the beating heart of yoga, as far as I'm concerned. Thank you for finding your way onto the mat. Thank you for standing with the group, stepping up for yourselves, and bringing your full attention to the practice of embodiment. There is so much to learn. I am humbled to share the path with people who invest so fully in the art of being human. I encourage you to keep exploring the patterns of whatever you are—whatever *we* are—in this wild and wonderful ocean of experience. It is a marvel to behold your work.

From Anthony

Thank you, Kyle, for your brilliant work as a teacher and writer. Thank you, Joyce Cellars, for your generous love and kindness. And thank you, Jazzy, Daphne, and Clio Cellars, for being so wonderful, *and* for occasionally napping at the same time (or visiting your gracious grandparents, Bethanne and Jeff) so that my part of this work could get done. Also, a huge thank-you to our editors at North Atlantic Books, Alison Knowles and Gillian Hamel, for their thoughtful attention to this project.

DEAR READER

Hello and welcome to this book. It's about yoga, sort of. Please don't get too excited. Behind this book's curtain is a (relatively) hairless monkey-thing who watches the movies and lets the dog lick all the way inside his ear-hole; who still occasionally bums cigarettes from the cool kids on restaurant patios and allows his own personal laundry to pile up, sometimes higher than he would allow guests to witness; whose excursions in the world have occasionally broken his brain a little bit.

This monkey is regularly confused by the lights and the not-lights all around him. "Where are the mangoes?" he asks, and he is pointed to a box of food so large he can climb his whole body inside of it. And then he can wander around the box's insides for hours on end. Often, he forgets why he is in the box, so he buys some Oreos. Word on the street is these Oreos are vegan, which is nice, because this monkey fancies himself an exceptionally compassionate wanderer of the giant food box.

There is still, for this monkey, a recurring desire to climb trees and howl at passersby. He lives in a loop of grooming, feeding, and screeching at the other monkeys about where the boundaries are and where they should be. Every now and then he pauses screeching, and closes his eyes for a while, and gets a few ideas about getting fewer ideas, which is a bit of a conundrum because he has discovered that counting ideas also counts as ideas. So, who knows?

Yoga shapes make this monkey a little less confused and a little more happy. So he spends much of his time doing yoga shapes and talking to other monkeys about being less confused and more happy and also about how sometimes things work and sometimes they don't. How sometimes things last for a while and sometimes they don't. The mangoes will sit on the counter for weeks until little black flies start circling and the monkey goes "fuck" and then the mangoes are tossed out the door in the bag. Nothing stays the same.

Of course, this monkey maintains a strange belief that he is different than, you know, monkeys. Sometimes he pretends his yoga shapes are turning him into a not-monkey. Sometimes he likes to think he is the first monkey that will never die. But he is not. The Oreos are delicious, and they are just Oreos. The mangoes taste sweet, and then, out with the bag. The yoga shapes are shapes like all the others.

So don't get too excited, because a mango is a mango and a breath is a breath. And behind this curtain is just a monkey-thing, like you, that is moving in shapes upon shapes in succession, one by one like the frames in those movies. And this monkey, like all monkeys, is watching to see what stories come out of the shapes. Because behind the movies, behind the frames, behind the shapes and the monkeys, and shining through all of the curtains, there is a light. And the light becomes the story.

INTRODUCTION

I took my first yoga class about seventeen years ago, but it didn't really stick. I was in college and, although I liked the class, I didn't have the motivation to establish a practice. I had other stuff going on. I truly "found" yoga when I was twenty-seven and I experienced Bikram Yoga for the first time. I was in a pretty dark place in my life at the time, and the safety and routine of the hot room became a stabilizing force. Also, I was—and am—a profusely sweaty person. When I was there, fathoms deep in a mirrored ocean of fire and spandex, soaking my yoga mat was not a sign that I was gross or repulsive; it was a mark of accomplishment. Heat transmuted my embarrassment into pride, reformed my idea of myself, and changed my life. I get the appeal.

Over the years, I took the opportunity to really dig into Bikram as a physical practice. I have taught thousands of classes and countless students how to perform Standing Bow and Fixed Firm and the like. I have advocated for the fundamental value of "26 and 2," as the sequence is known, and promoted practices like knee locking and depth seeking. However, I eventually encountered what felt like a fatal flaw in the Bikram Yoga world: there was almost no professional development available for me beyond the initial teacher training. I'm kind of a nerd, I like information, and I wanted to be the best teacher I could, so I branched out to see what else was out there. I studied widely, got certified in alternative styles, read a bunch of books, and soon came to discover that a lot of what I'd been teaching as undeniable Truth was suspect, or even directly contrary to current best practices.

This book, and the practice you will find within, is in many ways the result of this exploration. My initial aim in developing this method was to create a more functional hot yoga practice, an evolution of the "original" hot yoga style. However, as we will discuss toward the end of the book, the more I allowed myself to evolve, the less I believed hot yoga of any kind can be morally justified fully in the modern world.

That's a big statement. I get it. Maybe you'll agree with me, maybe you're already dousing this book in kerosene. You get to make your own choices. I'm going to present my case; the rest is up to you.

On Scandal

Any book even halfway related to the world of Bikram[1] would be incomplete without acknowledging the ongoing sex scandals involving Bikram Choudhury. This book is not a work of investigative journalism; it's mostly about bodies, but I won't minimize the destructive impact these scandals have had on individuals and communities both. Please do not interpret my focus on bodywork as an attempt to ignore these issues.

For me, I have no firsthand knowledge of Choudhury's salacious and hurtful behavior, so I will not attempt to insert myself into the conversation with any authority. All I'll say is, as a person who spent weeks around him in training, I believe his accusers. And the accusations are terrible. I must admit that though the reports of impropriety and assault made me angry, they didn't exactly surprise me. The Bikram persona that I experienced seemed explicitly self-centered and arrogant, and he had no qualms about both humiliating his students and complimenting their sexual appeal.

I can't prove anything; I wasn't in the room for any of the alleged events, but as a former member of the teaching community I have seen and heard enough to make up my own mind. And I have had to confront difficult questions about my participation in a system of harm. This has humbled me, and made me reflect on the capacity of devoted groups of humans to elevate and validate authority figures beyond their rightful place.

Yoga is powerful. It touches us on a deep level, and this power can be warped when we do not acknowledge our own psychological

---

[1] "Halfway related" is a pretty good way to describe things here, in my opinion.

vulnerability. One of the big lessons of the last fifty years of yoga is that guru types, especially male guru types, can manipulate the power of yoga for their own personal gain. And, in an important way, their corrupting influence indicts their followers. I look at my own participation in this apparently corrupt process with regret and shame, and have built my own path forward with as much intention as possible.

Yoga for Human Beings

The practice in this book is something I affectionately refer to as "Yoga for Human Beings." In many ways, this whole book is built on this platitude. I'm well aware the idea of "Yoga for Human Beings" is sort of redundant. By their report, when my editor presented this concept to their team, the group apparently asked, "Who else would yoga be for?" And that, my friend, is an excellent question. Unless the flamingos are doing it in secret or something, only human beings practice yoga.

In many ways this idea is a response to a sort of spiritual perfectionism I have encountered in the yoga community, particularly in the realm of marketing and stretchy pants and whatnot. Our culture manufactures a deluge of imagery and messaging about becoming and attaining and ascending, which are advertising techniques for making people feel like they're not quite good enough and should probably buy a tank top to reach their full potential. The story goes that the tank top is magical. Can't you tell? Look, the model in the tank top is smiling and putting a surfboard on top of a classic SUV on the side of the Pacific Coast Highway. Don't you want to be them?

The problem, of course, is the person in the ad isn't a human being. I mean, sure, the model is a human being. But the character in the ad is not human. That's just a story. Unfortunately, we are immersed in these kinds of stories so completely that they can begin to affect the way we think about ourselves in the world.[2]

---

[2] Some sources estimate modern human beings in the developed world see four thousand–plus advertisements a day. Ron Marshall, *Marketing Survival in a Digital World* (Springfield, MO: Big RAM, 2013), 17, cited in Red Crow Marketing, September 15, 2015, https://tinyurl.com/yyn5eogl.

Sadly, yoga is not immune to the market pressures of our current age. (Everybody's gotta make a living, right?) If you look around the yoga world, you'll sometimes find an implication that yoga practice is the work of turning into a character from an advertisement. This isn't always intentional, but it is encoded into the language we speak in this society. We have little aphorisms and platitudes and guidelines and images that constitute what it means to be a "good person," and they worm their way deep into our brains.

My own term for the characters from yoga advertisements is "sparkly perfect angel yoga people" or "SPAYPs."[3] The biggest issue with their existence is they give us this weird idea that we should act like them, look like them, eat like them, and aspire to their angelhood. But you're no angel, friend. Me neither. You're a human being. And like me you've got smelly intestines and bony tentacles and you experience the visual splendor of reality through orbs of jelly embedded in holes in your head. Part of what makes humans so wonderful is how weird and varied and fallible they are.

The point is, this is not Yoga for Angels. This is Yoga for Human Beings, here and now, in a challenging world.

On Cultural Appropriation

Yoga's path into the modern West has been a sort of wild ride. It encompasses a dark history of colonialism, the integration of Western fitness into traditional Indian spiritual practices, the evangelism of various teachers who first brought Eastern philosophy and then asana from India to the West, the rise of New Age ideas and white teachers, the scandalous fall of many (male) guru types, and the broad commodification of an ancient religion. Yoga is both an incredible gift to humankind and one of the world's premier examples of cultural appropriation. It can be a challenge to figure out how to embrace this gift without denigrating it.

---

[3] I have never actually used this acronym before.

There exists an undeniable tension between the profound benefit yoga has provided and continues to provide, and the reality that in the West the practice has been taken over, in large part, by affluent white people. I'm not going to try to resolve this tension. Its sociological and historical implications are daunting and beyond my expertise. And I'm not here to speak for a culture that isn't mine.

So, here's the full disclosure: I am not from India, nor is any member of my family as far back as I can tell. In fact, my sister once did one of those DNA tests, and it turns out that we are Anglo-German back as far as the genetic map can see. I don't claim to be an authority on traditional philosophy or Indian culture. I will dive into traditional concepts at about a seventh-grade level, to get us into a broader conversation about bodies and our place in the world. But I ain't a guru or a sage or a rishi. I'm inconsistent with both meditation and vegetarianism. As I write this, I'm on my third cup of coffee for the day. So, you know, take all traditional philosophy you find here with a grain of salt.

In terms of this book, I am using the word *yoga* in the broadest sense. In my experience, the modern definition of yoga in the West is a little slippery. We sometimes try to contain it with aphorisms like "yoga means union" but that's an oversimplification.[5] Again; I'm not going to try to resolve this matter, largely because it's not my place to do so.

---

[5] "Union" isn't really a complete translation. *Yoga* comes from the Sanskrit root *yuj,* which means "to yoke," like an ox to a cart. Which, yes, creates a form of union, but that's not the entire story. Depending who you ask, this can be either a comprehensive definition or a fairly useless one. I like it; it allows for a broad range of interpretations that leave room to explore, but I don't claim it's the "true" meaning or whatever. I've heard more traditional teachers define yoga as a form of science, or a preparation for meditation, with little regard for the "yoga means union" aphorism. Basically, there's no consensus definition of the word *yoga* that fits and fully honors every one of the myriad practice styles present in the world today. Or at least I haven't found one. To me, this conversation recalls what Supreme Court Justice Potter Stewart said in 1964 about the definition of pornography: "I know it when I see it." I'm not comparing yoga to pornography, but it does sometimes feel like our cultural definition of yoga follows similar logic: we know it when we see it.

I will focus not on what yoga means in a traditional sense, but more on the way it is spoken and heard in contemporary Western culture. I will spend little[6] time reflecting on the historical roots of yoga or traditional practices. Instead, I want to look at where we are, what we're working with, and how we can evolve. For the most part, yoga in the West is apparently a blend of bodywork, therapy, community, and occasionally a little bit of church. This book is primarily about the bodywork part; it's centered around human bodies as material things in a material world.

I will briefly explore a few traditional concepts in this book—namely *karma, tantra, samskara,* and *maya*—in an effort to demonstrate the link between ancient insight and present-day science. My aim is not to claim these concepts as my own but to celebrate the legitimacy and brilliance of the traditional philosophies of India. For I do find them brilliant. I will leave a more comprehensive exploration of these philosophies to others. My hope is that, should you be inspired by these ideas, you seek out further education from people more closely connected to the cultures that gave them life.

Origin Story

The method you are about to encounter is a synthesis, with input from modern bodywork methods, fitness styles, and physical philosophies. I encourage you to consider that synthesis is fundamental to the history and development of yoga. Indeed, many of the first yoga methods to become popular in the Western world borrowed heavily from European gymnastics exercises.

The key to the evolution of the Foundations of Repatterning, the method described in this book, is an emphasis on present-day human needs. It was built on the basic insight that human beings in the twenty-first century have issues that are unique to our time. To meet these unique challenges, we should seek the best information available. Some of the most creative and intelligent people in the world of bodywork are physical therapists (PTs), weightlifters, massage therapists, and the like.

---

[6] Read: "no."

Yoga is a container of sorts. It presents an opportunity to engage our bodies and minds within established boundaries. But how we fill this container is available for exploration. I haven't considered any particular yoga pose or command to be sacred. Instead, I have attempted to fill the container provided by the practice with a current understanding of the way humans move (or don't) in the present day.

So, some things may be familiar and some things may not. Some things may violate a sense of what is sacred to you; I hope you don't take it personally. I only ask that you hear me out, explore the information, and decide for yourself if this sort of approach resonates with you.

How to Read This Book

My sincere hope is that you find this thing enjoyable. To paraphrase *Mean Girls,* "I'm not a regular yoga book; I'm a cool yoga book."

While you'll probably get the most benefit from going through this thing in sequence, I've done my best to make it easy to read in random sections. Personally, I really like it when you can open a book to page 85 for no reason, read for ten minutes with no context, and walk away feeling like you've gained something valuable. I've aimed for that. Dive in at random places if you want, check out one section at a time, read it backward like *manga;* it's your call.

I've added a lot of "inserts" throughout, to help us branch out and explore the greater implications of the content (and to keep you disoriented so you never question the material too much). I have also drenched the entire text in high-grade early millennial sarcasm. In an effort to keep the main body of this thing flowing, I have relegated many of my worst attempts at humor to the footnotes.[7] If you're not a footnote person, or you just want to avoid some of the snark, you can skip them entirely. None of the essentials are down there; it's just citations, asides, and incidental information.

---

[7] Getting this in before you can: Yes, I read a lot of David Foster Wallace in my twenties. Yes, I took far too much pride in finishing *Infinite Jest.* Yes, I know he used endnotes and not footnotes in that one. No, he's not my most favorite author of forever and all time. (George Saunders, FTW.)

The main body of this book is part practice manual, part investigation of ideas. I have used many of the poses as jumping-off points for broader conversations beyond asana. I have generally tried to avoid anatomy lessons—there are other and far better sources out there for that kind of thing—though in some instances a short dive into the particulars will be necessary to serve the larger point.

If you are interested in more detailed information on human anatomy, check out the Recommended Reading (appendix 3) for book suggestions. You can also find breakdowns of the practice sequence in appendix 1, including half-hour, one-hour, and 75–90-minute versions of the class. Likewise, you'll find a condensed version of various guidelines and practice "rules" there.

Overall, my aim is to present a general practice theory, in service of a particular physical perspective. However, because I just can't contain myself, you'll find that our discussion will regularly breach the levees of bodywork and spill over into more expansive territory. OK. Away we go.

PART 1

YOGA FOR
HUMAN BEINGS

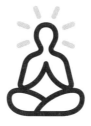

ON EVOLUTIONARY DESIGN

ere's a fun question: What are human beings? When we strip away our cars and our devices and our late-night adult cartoons, what exactly are we? I love this question, because at first it feels kind of simple—*a human being is a human being, dude, quit being weird and go pick up the Chinese food*—but when you dig into it things start getting a little slippery. Is a human being a bodysuit for a soul? Or maybe is the soul the "human" part? Are souls a thing at all? Am I just a meat robot? An illusion? An avatar in a video game? Who's steering this ship, anyway? Some of my favorite yoga teachers are the ones who play with this question, illuminating the nuance of experience by exposing assumptions and illusions. Like most things, the way you answer this question depends on the way you choose to see the world.

In yoga classes, we are sometimes asked to see the world through the lens of spirituality, or mythology, or emotion, or the cycles of nature. These are all wonderful perspectives to explore, each valid in its own way. However, they don't really help us out much when it comes to stuff like the anatomy of movement. Movement happens in the material world, and the best tools for understanding the material world are things like physics and chemistry and biology. These fields of study don't do much for us when we are searching for abstract metaphors that describe the indescribable, but they're great when we want to figure out why your spine has curves and your heart rate increases under stress.

If we are going to work with human beings, particularly their bodies and movement, it is vital that we understand the basics of evolution and natural selection. Which is fine; these basics are not so complex. Essentially, all life on earth has been in a certain way "designed" by death. If an organism could escape death long enough to reproduce, it succeeded in the game of natural selection, a game that combines environmental fitness with a hefty slice of random chance. (Not to be confused with the game of Snakes and Ladders, which is played exclusively by random chance and is hardly a game at all when you really think about it.) In order to win this game, an organism would benefit greatly from two advantages: efficiency and adaptability.

Efficiency means, in this case, that the organism doesn't spend any more energy than it has to survive. You spend too much energy, you need too much food, you starve. So living things have an evolutionary pressure to use no more energy than absolutely necessary to survive.[8] Not an evolutionary pressure to get shredded for swimsuit season or to actualize our dreams—to survive. Keep this in mind, it'll change everything when we talk about yoga poses.

Adaptability in this case means an organism or species can change to meet the needs of its environment. Sometimes this adaptation is long-term: it occurs over the course of many generations, like the evolution of opposable thumbs. Sometimes it's faster, like when you learn how to start a fire with a magnifying glass. When we do asana work, we are working directly with our capacity for (relatively) fast adaptation. Our ability to get stronger or more flexible is a form of adaptation. Our capacity to learn mindfulness and stress-relief through breathing—these are forms of adaptation too. In many ways, yoga is the practice of manipulating adaptation.

---

[8] Some species have figured a way around this. Porcupines, for example, are dull and lazy and almost entirely clueless wastes of space and tree bark. Which is fine for them because their skin is a hellish bed of nightmare death needles, and predators for such quarry are scarce.

Now, from this perspective, we ask again: What are human beings?

Human beings are bipedal primates. We have the most complex brains in the world, as far as we can tell. We are fundamentally social; we work together very well, which partly explains how we outlasted—and killed—larger and more powerful animals throughout our history. We thrive on almost every continent and in nearly every single terrestrial climate on earth. In other words, we are ridiculously good at adaptation.

Humans are well suited for a variety of physical activities, though there are a few in particular that are right in our wheelhouse: walking, running, swimming, climbing, throwing, carrying, and squatting. In fact, we are earth's champions at throwing. No organism is better at hurling projectiles through space, and it's really not even close.

We are also master runners. Yes, a cheetah or a gazelle would own a human being in an eight-hundred-meter race, but over marathon distances, human beings are nearly unmatched. Our two-legged stride, with an upright torso and powerful leg muscles, is hyperefficient for (relatively) medium-speed running. We use a twisting motion between the hips and ribs, plus a swing in the arms, to maximize power and minimize effort while covering long distances. Our labyrinthine and damp sinuses both purify and heat air when we inhale, so oxygen can be more easily integrated into our bloodstream. And our downward-facing nostrils keep our sinuses from drying out while we run. We're made for it.

Likewise for walking. Many early human beings were generally nomadic. We did a lot of wandering, even more than that one cousin of yours with the bracelets and the sandals and the blog. We can—and arguably *should*—walk for miles and miles on a regular basis. While "civilized" human beings are often limited by pain (knees, back, neck, etc.), it is difficult to imagine Paleolithic humans suffering from mass epidemics of walking-induced knee pain. We just wouldn't have survived. We needed to walk, and we did. A lot. And well.

The Modern Myth likes to pretend that we overcame the need for things like running and walking because we overcame the *material* need for them. Once we didn't need to run or walk for food, the Myth implies there kind of ceased to be a real point to it at all. Running is unnecessary, the Myth goes, and climbing is for kids, and swimming is a luxury, and throwing is reckless, and … are you really squat-sitting in public? This is a Walgreens! You don't need that stuff, the Myth whispers, and anyway, aren't you tired?[9] And we reply, Yes! I am tired. So nice of you to ask-slash-manifest that, Myth. I will not swing from the branches. Who has energy for such silly things?

But the Modern Myth is way off mark. What we're figuring out after years of easy living—processed food and suburban housing and micro-waves and the Country Music Awards—is that the things we evolved to do are the very same things that keep us healthy. We evolved to eat a variety of local plants and nuts, cooked food, and organic berries.[10] Those things keep us healthy, physically and emotionally. We evolved to live closely with other humans in the service of a common good. Our social groups define how we construct meaning and value. We evolved to walk and run; walking and running keep us healthy. You get the energy to run, in part, by running. This is your evolutionary design.

Now, I know what you're thinking: Dude, if you love running and walking and swimming and climbing so much, why do you teach yoga? Literally none of those things happen in a yoga class. You make an excellent point, Todd (can I assume your name is Todd?), and it brings us to our next idea, which has to do with connection, shapes, and the value of contradictory perspectives.

---

[9] There is an opposite but equally destructive myth out there, which we might call "Athleisure." That myth tells you that you should work out all the time, every day, because that's what good people do. Fashionable people. Worthwhile people. People with disposable income.

[10] "Organic" of course being an absurd term with regard to human beings who lived before pesticides and whatnot.

ON TRIBES

Here's a fun tidbit: the size of a primate's brain is directly related to the size of their social group.[11] Humans have the largest brains of all primates. We didn't get all big-brainy because we had an evolutionary pressure to invent power drills; we got this way largely because it helped us coordinate socially. We aren't snow panthers: we don't wander alone our entire lives, only meeting briefly to mate once every year or so. We're like wolves, or elephants. We're built to be part of a team.

And this design, this way we are made, shapes our well-being. Just like sitting on the couch for a week straight will make you feel terrible, so too will a week of zero human interaction. Connection is essential to our health.

Another part of the Modern Myth is that human beings construct meaning as individuals: that we are isolated nuggets of determination and responsibility and we all need to figure things out for ourselves. Good people, according to the Myth, "pull themselves up by their own bootstraps" and "forget what other people think" and are "ahead of the pack" and "stand out from the crowd" and all of the other advertising jargon.

This mentality, that we should think of ourselves as distinct units without any true connection to the people around us, doesn't benefit human beings. Largely because it's wrong, just like telling people they should eat ten Big Macs a week is wrong. This mentality does, however, help sell shampoo and discourage labor unions.

Please hold while Kyle takes a breath to collect himself so as to not turn this whole book into a rant about late-stage capitalism. ... elevator music ... OK, we're back.

Here's a thought experiment: what do you find most meaningful in your life? Family? Love? Art? Activism? Work? Competition? Religion? Practice? Odds are, you derive your greatest sense of meaning from something that

---

[11] Dunbar's number.

involves or benefits other human beings,[12] probably both. Other people are essential to our well-being. This isn't a glitch; it's part of your design. Don't let anyone tell you that you don't need people. You need people like you need protein, because you're a tribal animal. Even the most introverted and shy human beings regularly desire connection with others.[13] We evolved to work together just like we evolved to run or eat greens. What I'm saying is, working with and for other people is what makes life rich and meaningful, it makes us thrive.

Say it with me: cooperation is the new kale.

---

[12] Some people seem to have rewired this evolutionary system to derive meaning and well-being from a connection with cats or decorative plants. Like I mentioned, humans are remarkably adaptable.

[13] Barring, of course, pathological conditions, which are by definition outliers.

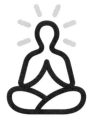

THE JOSEPHINE

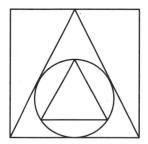

P op quiz, hotshot: What is this image? If you're the sort that likes abstract iconography or art theory, you might come up with all kinds of ideas. It's a mountain or a shrine, maybe. Or maybe it's the Eye of Ra. Perhaps it's a representation of the struggle of the inner child to manifest the heart's desires within an oppressive superstructure, the soft curving feminine desperate to escape the prison of masculine vertical triangles that staunchly uphold the "square" mentality of cultural orthodoxy. Maybe it's a goose. Who knows? You can choose. You can make this image mean whatever you want. That's part of the beauty of being human.

But before all that: for a moment let's forget the idea of image as representation or symbol and just look at it from a clean slate. What is it? How could we describe it? Imagine I'm seven years old, tell me what you see.

Odds are you're thinking something like, "it's a square with a triangle inside of it. There's a circle inside the triangle and a smaller triangle inside the circle." You are absolutely correct, that's precisely what it is. From a certain perspective.

When we look at this image we see it the way we have been *trained* to see it. We see four shapes in one image because long ago when we were very young we learned about each of these individual shapes, partially because they're so simple. They're wired into our unconscious brains like language or the lyrics to "Gangsta's Paradise,"[14] so most of us look at the image and see triangle-circle-triangle-square. These simple distinct shapes define the image; it exists as their combination.

But what if we looked at it another way? What if we looked at the image as one unified shape? A much more complex shape than we're used to, sure, but just one shape nonetheless. It's not four things together; it's just one thing. And if it's just one thing, it needs a name, because if we keep on calling it "the image," we'll never shake the voice inside chanting "triangle-circle-triangle-square." So we will call this image a Josephine.

A Josephine is its own shape. Sure, the easiest way to describe it would be to say "it's a triangle in a circle in a triangle in a square." But that's not really what it is, because it's a Josephine. It's all one thing. Every time you try to bend the square border on a proper Josephine, the triangles and the circle bend too. If you try to "smush" a Josephine like a spring, every line and shape respond, smushing along with it. This is because the Josephine is not actually a triangle in a circle in a triangle in a square. It's a Josephine.

When we are studying Josephines, we have to be careful, because a triangle expert might come along someday and say, "Hey, those are triangles right there. Those triangles are important. Let me tell you about their three sides and the stability of their structure and how the sum of their interior angles is always 180 degrees." And the triangle expert, because he's smart and well-meaning and probably has an advanced degree in triangles, will make a very convincing argument that the most important part of a Josephine is those embedded triangles. And we will likely all

---

[14] They say I've got to learn, but nobody's here to teach me.

believe him. But then a circle expert will show up and revolutionize the Josephine field, pointing out the nuance and brilliance of a perfect circle. And she will make an equally convincing argument that true understanding of a Josephine requires a circle-first approach.

And they will both have really good points. Neither one would be wrong. A deep knowledge of circles and triangles (and squares) will undoubtedly deepen our understanding of a Josephine, but we can't forget the big picture. We have to keep in mind that a Josephine is more than a combination of shapes. A Josephine is its own shape.

What we have now are two perspectives for understanding the Josephine:

1. The composite view: a Josephine is what we call a composition of simple, distinct elements. In this view it is best described as a "triangle in a circle in a triangle in a square."

2. The holistic view: a Josephine is the (recently made-up) name of a single complex shape.

Very important to note, here. Neither of these views is necessarily right. Their contradiction should not be mistaken for debate. These are simply two different ways to think, both valid in their own way. As students we want to honestly engage both perspectives. That's how we'll really figure out the Josephine, looking at it from different angles of the mind.

OK, but WTF

At this point you may be squinching one eyeball a bit. That's reasonable. Why did we just do this? Why did we invent a Josephine for a yoga book?

Well, let's play a game. Look at your hand. It's all right: this particular book was specifically designed to remain fully operational during one-handed use. Hold your hand out in front of you and take a moment to really investigate it. How would you describe your hand? Use the simplest terms imaginable. What would you say?

You're likely conjuring words like "fingers" and "knuckles" and "nails" and "skin." If you're getting anatomical, you're maybe thinking of metacarpals and capillaries, stringy tendons and smooth bursae. When you describe your hand this way, as fingers and knuckles, muscle and tendon, you're using the composite view. You've broken the hand into hand-pieces, like breaking a Josephine down into shapes. And this is great. This is useful. This is how we make complicated stuff like hands or the weather or Aussie rules football make sense: we take them apart into pieces because the entire phenomenon is mind-bogglingly complex.

However, your hand is not just a composite of simple parts; it's also a complex whole. Sure, it's a bunch of tendons and muscles and skin and bone, but it's also a hand. And even your hand is just a component of your arm, which is a component of your whole body.

Try this. Make your hand into a fist. Squeeze that fist real hard. Hard as you can. Now, holding that fist, feel what's happening in your elbow. You will notice that there's a lot of tension in your elbow when you make a fist. That's not because your elbow is part of your hand, per se. It's because you don't have a hand, or rather you don't have a hand in isolation. (By the way, you can release that fist now.)

The trouble, with bodies as with Josephines, shows up when we get stuck. When we forget to see the whole image, we become hypnotized by the simplicity of the component parts. And the hypnosis of simplicity is far more seductive than most of us realize. We actually have a psychological bias toward simplicity. Our brains *love* simple stuff, and when they think they've found it, they hold on with both hemispheres. Our mental lives are filled with components, little pieces of the greater whole that we use to comprehend the world. For the most part, we don't even notice we have manifested these pieces at all.

This idea, that your hand does not exist as an isolated component, is vital to an honest investigation into the way that our bodies operate. Bodies, it turns out, aren't cleanly divided into pieces. "Body parts" are, for the most part, just our brain's way of making something unfathomably complex as simple as possible. For example: you do not have muscles. Of course, you have muscles. But you also don't have muscles. You have patterns.

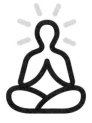

ON PATTERNS

One of the wonderful insights yoga provides us is the truth of interconnectedness. We are woven together. The word *tantra* literally means "loom" in Sanskrit, as in the thing that weaves tapestries and rugs. Every individual strand of creation is woven into the comprehensive whole. A change at one point in the system ripples and reverberates throughout its entirety. The ongoing, ceaseless interplay of these infinite ripples across space and time manifests as what we call "reality" or "the universe" or "all the stuff."

This becomes important when we start to look at movement. Human bodies are not made up of distinct individual parts; they are comprehensive wholes. You are, in a way, woven together. So everything is in constant interaction, influencing and reacting to everything else around it. This might sound complex, but when you boil it down it sounds something like: *The hip bone connected to the … thigh bone … the thigh bone connected to the … knee bone …*

Think for a moment about your hamstrings, right there on the back of your thigh. They don't operate in isolation; they have a cooperative relationship with your quads and your calves and your glutes, to name a few. Even when the hamstrings fire in isolation, without, say, the calves, this action is fundamentally defined by the inactivity of surrounding structures. If your calves and hamstrings fire together, you get one action. If they don't, you get another. Either way, these adjacent muscles inform one another because they are part of an integrated whole. Coexistence means cocreation, regardless of the balance of power. So, while in one way you have individual muscles and muscle groups, in another way you don't, because no physical action happens in isolation.

When you walk you don't just move your legs, you move your whole body. Your arms swing; your back and core muscles respond and interact to keep you upright and help coordinate rotation; your neck adjusts to balance your skull nicely on the top of your spine. Pick something, anything in your body—it's in the game.

Now, the *way* you walk—or stand, or run, or swim, or sit, whatever—is unique to you. You've got a unique body; where you're strong and weak, tight and loose, long and short, heavy and light, and to what degree, these things are all personal and singular. Your history, your injuries, your habits, and your genes all inform the way your body operates in the world.

For example, if you sprain your left ankle a bunch of times, the way you walk will start to shift. Scar tissue in your ankle will subtly change how your left foot lands, and your right foot will compensate. Your hips will adjust to accommodate this new movement, so your spine will adjust, so you'll carry your shoulders differently … you get the idea. I'm not saying that all of these adjustments will be major or apparently life-altering. They might not even be noticeable to you. Your body does a lot of stuff without "informing" you.[15]

The sum total of all of these adjustments—adaptations—creates what we will call a "pattern." We might say that this particular example is a "left ankle sprain pattern." You have countless other patterns within the system of your body as well. Some of them are the result of your past actions and some are the result of your genes. If you ride a bike, you'll

---

[15] For example; right now your pituitary gland is responsible for keeping, like, 89 percent of your shit together, and that thing will send you straight to voicemail every single time you call.

likely have a "cycling pattern" (strong thighs, shoulders forward). You might have a genetic pattern for wide hips, which will change how you walk. If you sleep on your belly, you might have a "head turned to one side pattern." You might have all of the above. Altogether, these countless patterns layer together to create an overall body pattern.

Your body pattern carries the sum total of all of your past actions. Every action you have ever performed is somehow practiced into you. Every time you climbed the stairs, you patterned "stairs" into your body. Every time you looked up at the stars, you patterned "stargaze" into your system. The more you practiced any particular action, the more deeply it patterned into your body, and the less effort and focus it required. Like your brain and speech organs learn a language, your body learns movement. The more you do it, the less you have to think about it.

KARMA AND SAMSKARAS

The word *karma* literally means "action" in Sanskrit. Philosophically, karma ties closely to the law of causation—the understanding that past events inform and shape present conditions, which then define the future.[16] This idea can sometimes feel a little exotic, but in many ways it's right in line with our understanding of human bodies (including our brains). When you play a game of tennis, the actions you take—backhand, forehand, lunge—are imprinted onto you, both mentally and physically. Your brain changes to create memory and integrate your experience. Your body changes in response to the demands for power and movement the game imposed. The past—your game of tennis—literally *becomes part of you*. What's more, the *way* that you played that

---

[16] To some degree. How much the future is "determined" by past conditions is the subject of endless debate and gets pretty wild the more you dig in. Which isn't to warn you off; wild can be great. Just … you know … bring a helmet.

game of tennis was not only informed by every tennis game you played before, but also by every single action you've ever taken in your entire life. Every step, every drink, every evening in front of Netflix, everything from the past informed that tennis game. And now that tennis game has changed you too.

In terms of cosmology, the Law of Karma embraces this concept right down to the essence of reality. "Now" carries the patterns of the eternal "then" inside of it, acts according to their influence, and then enters into them as time moves on.

There's an interesting extension to this spiritual perspective that aligns with modern brain science and psychology: Samskaras.[17] Broadly defined, samskaras are deeply ingrained patterns in the mind (or spirit? It's a tough distinction in this context) that affect us deeply and guide our behavior in the world. They are often hidden from our conscious mind, but they have a profound effect on our behaviors and experiences. You might imagine a captain guiding his ship across a broad ocean, unaware the vessel is tethered to a Leviathan in the deep. He can turn the wheel and rig the sails, but if he does not acknowledge and compassionately train[18] the Leviathan, he will never fully be in charge.

If we are to grow, it is helpful to know what our deepest illusions are, as they inform our perspectives, our identities, and our daily emotions. The field of neuroscience has discovered that our most common thoughts and feelings—like the ones we have about ourselves and our vital relationships—create the most well-established neuronal connections in the brain. These strong connections are sometimes called "core beliefs." Such beliefs are embedded deep in our unconscious mind, encoded onto the lower two

---

[17] The literal Sanskrit definition for *samskara* is "activator."

[18] PSA: Negative reinforcement training is not advised when working with elemental creatures and mythological archetypes.

levels of our triune brain: the brainstem and limbic system.[19] In a way, this is our Leviathan, our deepest genetic and historical karma, hidden beneath the surface yet still powerful. And the more we let this creature guide the ship, the stronger it becomes.

Luckily, the revelation of neuroplasticity has taught us that our brains change in response to our daily lives. Literally, every thought, action, and experience we have changes the patterns in the physical structure of our brains. And these patterns fundamentally inform our thoughts, actions, and experiences.

Patterns inform actions that inform patterns. Samskaras inform karma which informs samskaras. Isn't yoga awesome?

---

[19] The limbic system, the second of the three layers of your brain, is usually what we're talking about when we mention the "lizard brain." It handles the fight, flight, freeze, feed, fear, fornicate part of life. The third layer of the triune brain is your neocortex, which is responsible for higher conscious functions like logic, problem solving, and abstract thought. The activity of the neocortex is normally what human beings identify as the "self." We are not just the captain; we are the Leviathan as well.

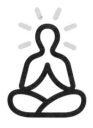

REPATTERNING

For each and every one of us, there are grooves of behavior that we slide into easily, thoughts we return to over and over, places where we're constantly tense, muscle groups that always seem to seize up, and on and on. We call them habits, and they are dominant forces in our daily lives. As much as we might like to think of ourselves as independent agents who constantly make choices throughout the day, human beings are actually pretty predictable. Habits, patterns in our behaviors, fundamentally inform the process of our lives.

Yoga helps us interact with our habits by first slowing us down to investigate them, then injecting a new (arguably super-weird?) set of behaviors into our lives. These new behaviors, which in yoga are called practices, modify our mental and physical patterns. When we change our behavior, we change our bodies and minds. If we add a little intelligence and a lot of intention to this mix, we can start to reform the big picture of our lives. In this way, the ritual practice of yoga has a special power to gradually reorganize patterns of all kinds. In this book, we will call this process "repatterning."

> Repatterning: The process of intentionally modifying habitual patterns through intelligent, routine action.[20]

---

[20] Note that not all changes in body patterns fit our definition of repatterning. As far as we are concerned, repatterning is performed intentionally with a specific goal in mind.

In terms of physical practice, yoga repatterns the way your body holds tension. This is true of any physical activity, for sure, but yoga is somewhat unique in the area; it emphasizes repetition and dedication, a regular return to established postures, moderate intensity, and a willingness—indeed, usually a central edict—to slow down and pay attention.

Body patterns include every cell in your own personal organism. There's nothing left out. Nobody's got a rogue pancreas that refuses to be involved; the whole system interacts. However, as yoga students interested in how bodies move, we are primarily concerned with a few particular systems: muscles, connective tissue, and bone. Bone is determinative and very important to acknowledge, but it doesn't change its shape very much through practice (at least on the timescale we're talking about in this book.) Muscles inform body patterns by providing power. They adapt by gaining or losing strength and mass, which changes the way the body holds itself and moves around. The type of muscle fiber—fast-twitch or slow-twitch—can shift somewhat and affects movement as well.

Connective tissue is a fibrous network that distributes and coordinates tension throughout the body.[21] It includes ligaments and tendons, but extends far beyond these limited structures. It is interwoven throughout the body (remember tantra?) and wraps around nearly every other tissue in the body, muscles and organs, to help hold them in position.

In the practice of yoga we work with the capacity of this tissue to deform and adapt over time, which allows us to change our tension patterns. When we "stretch" a muscle and gain flexibility, the individual muscle fibers[22] must adapt and reform, which is vital to our capacity to generate force.

The way we use our practice to change tension patterns is up to us. What are our standards? Where are we going? How do we want our bodies to feel and move? If we are going to do the work of repatterning, it's important to define what exactly we are trying to achieve.

---

[22] Sarcomeres.

[21] Among lots of other stuff.

FUNCTIONAL MOVEMENT

The term "functional movement" has become a bit of a cliché in the fitness world, which bugs me to no end because I am a hipster and therefore allergic to popular things. But the standards of functional movement are a great way to investigate and interpret physical practices. For our purposes, we will define a "functional movement practice" as an activity that serves three main goals:

1. Diversity: Functional movement practices should support healthy movement across a wide spectrum of activity. The wider the better. This doesn't just mean you can move your limbs in all directions; it also means you can create power and stability when needed. Following the Rule of Three (as described in the following section), a functional practice embraces the relationship between mobility and strength to support the largest range of potential activity.

2. Longevity: Functional movement practices should create healthy movement patterns that do not destabilize or injure the body over time. If we achieve our goal of diversity but it only lasts for six months before starting to wear your body down, we should revise our practice.

3. Relevance: Diversity and longevity will be deeply informed by the needs and desires of the students performing the practice. If you live in a location where the floor is lava, we should tailor your diversity toward nimble movement, grip strength (for the vines), and balance. If you live in a dystopian future where everybody is held to the ground with magnet shoes, functional practice should emphasize quad strength.

In our definition, functional movement practices are not self-referential, meaning they don't aim specifically to reinforce themselves. In self-referential practices the primary aim is to improve your skill at that practice. For example, shooting a basketball is self-referential; you shoot a basketball to get better at shooting a basketball. Physical therapy is not self-referential. When you do PT exercises you are trying to make your body more functional for activities that are not themselves PT.

While yoga is well-suited to fit the mold of functional movement, there is also a tendency for students to make yoga a self-referential practice. The postures can become both the practice and the goal, the means and the end. For example, if you're practicing back bends just so you can be "better" at back bending, you might lose sight of the functional purpose of their practice. (Or you just might not care about the functional value of the practice, which is your right. You get to choose what you want.) The Foundations of Repatterning, the practice we will soon learn, is intentionally built from the ground up as a functional movement practice that is not self-referential. Its goal is not to make you "good at yoga"; it's to provide you with the basic tools you need to powerfully engage in the activities of your ongoing, wonderful human life.

SPIRITUAL PRACTICE AND FUNCTIONAL MOVEMENT

Yoga has significant value outside of the physical component of practice. To describe it in purely physical terms robs it of its depth. I'm not here to take sides about the specific metaphysical value of particular practices. Instead, I will ask you to entertain the notion that spiritual practice is not necessarily style-specific. (There are yoga teachers who may disagree with me on this, but I think the point should be aired out.)

We might consider that any particular spiritual approach can be infused into any physical practice. It's possible that we could play Kundalini Baseball. Or take a chakra-opening walk. These might not be the *best* physical activities for such spiritual practices, but that doesn't mean they're inherently *wrong* for them. We might entertain the idea that any physical action can serve as a vessel for any spiritual pursuit. (Lots of people do their deepest spiritual work sitting in chairs.) There is arguably nothing spiritually exclusive to yoga poses; yoga poses are just available—and potentially effective—vehicles for that sort of work.

I'm sort of taking some air out of "traditional" yoga postures here, but that's the point. I have seen many yoga teachers justify functionally unjustifiable practices with metaphysical or psychological concepts. (For example, I have repeatedly heard yoga teachers speak about hip openers as a sort of emotional or spiritual cleanse. We will get into this later when we talk about Pigeon, but needless to say, keeping your hips physically stable is vital to your long-term well-being. Extreme hip opening has the potential to damage those major joints and create maladaptive movement patterns.) I propose to you the idea that it is possible to build a practice that is first and foremost about physical concepts, like functional movement, and apply whatever spiritual or emotional or psychological ideas we choose on top of them. We are baking a cake together; you can decorate it however you like.[23]

---

[23] No walnuts, though.

Within our mission in this book, esoteric concepts like chakras or *nadis* or kundalini[24] don't determine the shape or style of the practice. Psycho-spiritual benefits, whatever they might be, aren't our central focus here. We're not leaning toward spiritual practice, nor are we leaning away. There's no leaning.

---

[24] These terms will not be on the test. Don't worry about it.

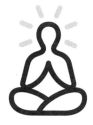

THE RULE OF THREE

Here's a completely implausible scenario that has certainly never happened to you, personally:

Somewhere in the unforgiving, dust-strewn desecration that is social media—that cackling wasteland into which we have all been cast with neither map nor guide—you encounter someone with whom you disagree. You disagree with them on a deep level and merely engaging with them has the potential to make you profoundly upset. We will call them your Nemesis.

Your Nemesis happens to post something about a current hot-button issue one day, with an accompanying opinion that you cannot stand. Like, your shoulders go into your neck just from reading it. For whatever reason you decide to engage your Nemesis in a debate. Maybe you want to make the world a better place; maybe you're overcaffeinated; maybe you just read a BuzzFeed article about all the ways people like your Nemesis is making the world worse. Who knows. You engage. The comment thread between you and your Nemesis really gets kicking, thousands of words flying across the digital ether, each argument more convincing than the last (yours, not theirs, of course). At some point you almost decide to throw up your hands and walk away and find a couch cushion to scream into. But then, out of nowhere, you notice something: your

Nemesis has made—deep in the weeds of a debate that is clearly no longer about the original topic—a decent point. Just one. Decent. Point. You can't deny it; there's something there.

And this makes you pause. It makes you reform and reorient and rethink a bit. You're not abandoning your principles, you're just—for a moment—forced to accept that someone so fundamentally opposed to you could be ... correct? And that you might, at least in this one instance, be wrong. Maybe for a moment you feel like your brain is short-circuiting. Maybe you hold your breath and screw up your face. If you're lucky, maybe all of the above.

And there, right there on the razor's edge between one idea and its opposite, where you're a little lost and hanging in midair? Where your certainty and the certainty of your Nemesis are at odds and the outcome is unknown? That's where the juice is. That's where things are interesting, valuable, and worth your time.

This is what we will call the Rule of Three:[25] There are three components to all vital interactions: a point, its counterpoint, and the relationship between them. For valuable experience—for the juice of reality—we need all three. The spark of life exists in the tension between opposites, not their resolution.

For example, light and dark. Easy peasy. If there were only light, we wouldn't have any shadow and shape, right? In essence, if there's only light, there's nothing. There's no definition, no contour, no interest. And if there were only dark, we'd have a nearly identical problem. The magic of visual experience happens in the meeting, the interplay of these opposites.

You can play this game with all dualities:

- good versus evil
- past versus future
- life versus death

---

[25] Not to be confused with the Rule of Three from writing and comedy, which is unrelated, irrelevant, and super-effective.

- individual versus community
- authority versus autonomy
- mental versus physical
- pleasure versus pain
- free will versus determinism
- getting truth across via Instagram versus Instagram is inherently evil

You get the idea.

In Western philosophy we might consider this as a form of Hegelian dialectic; one thing (thesis) interacts with its counterpoint (antithesis), and through this interaction, this conflict, we arrive at synthesis, a new kind of "truth" (or really, just the grounds for the next argument). In Eastern philosophy it's most clearly embodied by the yin-yang of Taoism, which illustrates the dance of opposites, reinforcing and driving one another, inseparable and polar at once.

I'll ask you now to recall the Sanskrit root of the word *yoga* is *yuj*, meaning "to yoke." Yoga—sometimes translated as "union" or "team"—can be explored as a manner of taking two things, like an ox and a cart, and binding them together.

What is important here is this "union" does not entail two things but three. You have a concept, its counterpoint, and their relationship. This relationship—the third point—is the conversation between dualities, and it is in this versatile and dynamic interaction that we gain insight. When we go too far to one side, the other side—the antithesis, or the yang, or whatever—will spring up to remind us we're missing something. A new conflict may emerge and demand that you pay attention, learn, and grow from the interaction.

Here's a pertinent example: there is a fairly well-known history of yoga gurus guiding students toward a sense of freedom and well-being, while also abusing and manipulating some of them. Both parts of this duality contain truth—some of these gurus do in fact teach interesting and valuable concepts—but they're rarely discussed in tandem. As long as one side or the other is repressed or overlooked, we fail to engage honestly with the full breadth of the situation. By engaging the complexity of these interactions—these conflicts—we may discover a more nuanced understanding of who and what we are.[26]

And in this engagement we are never "done."[27] This goose never gets cooked through. We often *want* to be done because then we could rest, comfortable in our correctness. If we are done, we're safe. We're stable. Indeed, "You are right, complete, blessed, pure, perfect, whole, the best" are all—in a sense—ways of saying "You are done." But unfortunately, direct and honest interaction with life doesn't work that way. Change will destabilize us all, over and over, because the game of life is about relationship, not resolution. A resolution is inert. It's death. If you ever find a total sense of resolution, it's time to go in search of an opposite.

Another way to say this is, solutions are overrated. We're wading into murky philosophical bayous here, but there's a good argument to be made that human beings are built for some degree of conflict. Having something to stand for or push back against is central to our well-being, if only because it provides us with a sense of purpose. It's encoded into our DNA. Recall that evolution is a dance, or a competition, with death. The hard truth is that if you want to eat, you have to eat other forms of life. Unblemished pacifism is not only unavailable, its pursuit denies nature.

I understand that these are rather grand pronouncements for a book about sweaty mammals and cell phones and connective tissue. I'll ask for your patience. My hope with this book is to take a few ideas apart, like a three-year-old with a screwdriver, and then maybe see if we can't put some new ones back together.

In physical terms, the Rule of Three is readily apparent. Understanding how bodies work involves understanding the value and function of opposites: rest versus work; agonist versus antagonist; inhale versus

---

[26] Fun to note: entertainment is almost universally an account of conflict between counterpoints. *Romeo and Juliet* would be a pretty lame play if their respective families were all like, "We totally support your decisions, kids!"

[27] Until we are.

exhale. Taking care of your body is not about resolving relationships but engaging in their ongoing complexity.

But we will see the rule elsewhere too. In fact, once you start to apply it, it pops up all over the place. In terms of the tension patterns of your body, we will explore the Rule of Three according to something we call Healthy Neutral; how can we balance the body evenly front and back? Side to side? Likewise, the relationship of mobility and stability is key to our practice. You can get too mobile. You can get too stable. As we practice yoga we intentionally shape these relationships.

Tension

Tension can get a bad rap in yoga classes. It's not too uncommon to hear talk about tension that associates it with chronic stress and anxiety. While there are some really interesting theories about the ways in which your body "stores" trauma and anxiety,[28] it is a dangerous oversimplification to make a direct connection between physical tension and negative emotions.

Tension is essential to every physical structure in the universe. If a structure doesn't have tension, it either disperses into entropy like stardust in interstellar space, or it collapses inward on itself like a neutron star. When planetary gravity gets involved, the importance of tension is even more apparent. Your skeleton is a major part of your human tension structure. It supports you against the pull of gravity. However, without the additional tension of muscles and connective tissue to support it, your skeleton would collapse in a heap. (You know those plastic human skeletons that some people use for anatomy lessons? They show up in yoga studios occasionally? Ever see one of those things standing up on its own? Nope. They all need an external structure to support them, because human skeletons aren't made to stand up on their own. Just like your muscles need bones to stay upright, your bones need your muscles, and connective tissue, etc.)

---

[28] See: pretty much everything Bessel van der Kolk has ever touched.

It's important we keep in mind that tension is not just good, it's *essential*. If we remove too much tension from our muscles and connective tissue surrounding the joints, the weight of the body can start to "sit" on or compress these joints; the "hard" structures have to compensate for tension that the "soft" structures aren't providing. Over time, this can be bad news for these joints. They are designed to work in tandem with balanced tension in the muscles and connective tissue, which helps create space between the bones and allows for smooth movement.

This isn't an argument for getting "tight" or never doing flexibility work. It's a call to mindful engagement of the practice. Remember the Rule of Three. We may benefit from removing a significant amount of tension from our bodies, but for each and every one of us there is the potential to go too far. A good way to think about it is, we want to ensure our bodies have access not just to relaxation, but also to balanced, well organized tension.

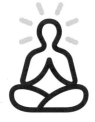

HEALTHY NEUTRAL

When our body patterns are in harmony with our evolutionary design, we are in a state we will call "Healthy Neutral." Healthy Neutral happens when the tension patterns in your muscles and connective tissue are well balanced and match the structure of your organs and bones. In the context of standing or sitting, Healthy Neutral is essentially "good posture." At the squat rack at the gym, it might be called "good form." We are seeking a more comprehensive definition that can be applied to yoga poses in service of functional movement.

Before we get too deep into this, we should be clear: Healthy Neutral is not a Platonic ideal; it's a map for the journey. There is no "perfect" or "correct" version of a human being. Humans are not built in a factory. We are natural things with loads of physical variation. That's good. We should celebrate that. Healthy Neutral doesn't show up the exact same way for every human. It will take mindful exploration for you to discover the way it shows up for you.

One way to find Healthy Neutral is to inspect our relationship with gravity in a standing position. Are we relatively even, forward and back? Side to side? Is our spine well-oriented with the hips, heart, and head in a general vertical line? Or are we twisted, leaning, or hunched?

Another way to evaluate Healthy Neutral is our alignment with evolutionary design. Are we well suited for basic human movements? Does it feel comfortable and natural to walk and run? To squat down? To climb over a boulder? To lift a child up on your shoulders? The actions that informed our evolution are still applicable today. We are still hairless primates. Natural selection did a wondrous job designing adaptable, efficient human bodies. While many factors—like age and injury—will determine how well we can move, we might consider that one way we get closer to freedom of movement is to get closer to Healthy Neutral.

We can, in this way, investigate some of the ways our context—modernity, civilization, pizza rolls, etc.—informs us. Have we maintained Healthy Neutral within and despite the overall change in human lifestyles? Or have we developed adaptations that are contrary to our well-being? Have we adapted a physical shape that doesn't move very well anymore?

We should take a moment here and remember: adaptation is generally a good thing. Humans become more efficient and well suited for their environment by developing and maintaining movement patterns that meet our daily needs. An Eskimo does not really need to have a palm-tree climbing pattern, but the harpoon-throwing pattern is probably nice to have. The wrist strength, the cross-body snap of the throwing arm, the steady position of the skull, the stability in the legs and rotation in the hips—all are necessary to effectively throw a heavy hunting spear, and all are practiced into the physical bodies of the humans who perform that action. Human adaptation kept us alive for thousands of years. It made us the dominant species and the apex predator on the planet. It helped give us culture, civilization, and yoga.

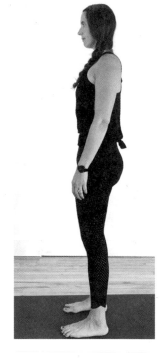

But now it's kind of off the rails.

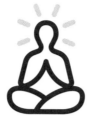

CHAIRS, FLOORS, SHOES, AND CELLS

I f you were to put a sling on your arm one day—for no good reason; you're not hurt—and wear it for about seven hours, your arm would feel pretty weird when you took it off. Your bicep would probably be tight; maybe your shoulder would be tweaky; you might find your hand a little less nimble than you like. But no big deal: after a minute or two of shaking your arm around like you're fighting off a swarm of bees, things would mostly get back to normal.

Now imagine that, starting at age four or five, you wore that sling for an extended period of time every single day of your life until right now. What do you think your arm would be like then?

Modern human beings, especially in the developed world, spend way too much time in chairs. We're talking a dangerous, frightening amount of time. Between six and ten hours on average *every single day*. And this happens early. It starts at preschool and only ramps up over time. Every day, millions of us train our bodies to adapt to chairs and couches and car seats. We learn from them and mold ourselves to fit their shape. Add in digital technology and cars and level floors everywhere, and we start to see some extraordinary adaptations. They often don't seem extraordinary, because so many people have them, but just because something is common does not mean it's healthy. On the contrary, many modern human beings have reshaped their bodies to suit a lifestyle that does not sync up with thousands of years of evolution. We have physically wrapped ourselves around modernity.

As with everything, the way any particular body responds to chair-bound modern life will be unique. However, there are some major body patterns that are common to many modern human beings.

1. Shoulder Hunch

Quick, find your cell phone. It's nearby, I'm sure. Now, sit down and hold your phone with both hands like you're about to send a text or play Candy Crush or something. OK, pause. What's going on right now with your shoulders?

It might sound weird because it's so obvious, but we primarily interact with the world in front of us. And when we sit down to work or text or whatever, we tend to round toward the object we're interacting with.

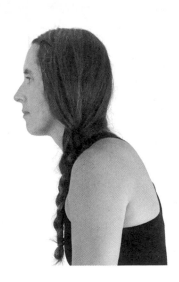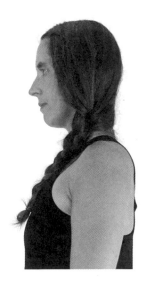

This rounding draws the shoulders forward of their "natural" neutral alignment. This is fine for a while, but if you do this a lot, then over time your body adapts and "learns" this pattern. The tissue in front of your shoulders—mainly your pectoral muscles and their associated connective tissue—tends to get shorter. The tissue of your upper back—mainly your rhomboids, upper lats, and lower traps, plus connective tissue—gets long.

In order to make this cell-phone, keyboard, book, or whatever position efficient, requiring less muscular energy, your body can grow patterns of connective tissue around this hunched shape. The muscles in your back then get weaker because they're not being used as much anymore, since their job is now being done by dense connective tissue. To reverse this, we need to build power in the upper back, and work on opening the top of the chest and fronts of the shoulders. When we do this effectively, the upper back muscles can hold our shoulders stable in healthy alignment, in line with the heart.

It's important to note that opening the front of the chest is not simply a matter of adding flexibility. If we do heart-opening exercises by themselves, we will be able to move the shoulders into a neutral position, but without corresponding strength in the back, we may not be able to maintain the position for long. To effectively balance the system, you need both: mobility and stability.

A healthy effective yoga practice should help to open the front of the chest while simultaneously strengthening the upper back.

2. Forward Head Carriage

Our forward orientation also shows up in the way we hold the skull at the top of the spine. When the body has a healthy plumb line, it holds the skull generally above the shoulders. However, in many modern settings—sitting in chairs, working at computers, looking at cell phones—we tend to push the skull forward of the shoulders.

Spend long enough in this position and the tissue behind your skull starts to adapt.[29] It can get stronger and tighter, in order to stabilize your skull toward the back of the neck. Meanwhile, in the front of the neck, the muscles get long and lose their strength.

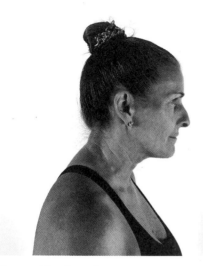

Forward head carriage.

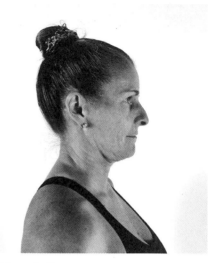

Neutral alignment.

---

[29] One fairly recent study from Australia highlighted some pretty wild consequences in young people who use phones a lot. Apparently, and this was just one study, so let's take it with a grain of salt, but apparently kids have been growing bony "horns" on the backs of their skulls from cell phone use (David Shahar and Mark G. L. Sayers, "Prominent Exostosis Projecting from the Occipital Squama More Substantial and Prevalent in Young Adult Than Older Age Groups," *Scientific Reports* 8:3354 (2018), doi:10.1038/s41598-018-21625-1). The theory goes, much like prolonged excess tension in the calf muscle can cause bone spurs on the back of the heel, prolonged excess tension behind the skull can give you, like, a bony rat tail. Let's not linger on this too long, yeah?

Try this. Lie down on your back on the floor and gently tuck your chin toward your chest, maybe just an inch or so, like you're giving yourself a double chin. Now float your head half an inch off the ground. Odds are, your chin will "want" to lift away from your chest, making the back of your neck shorter. If you resist this action, keeping the chin down, you may start to feel muscles in the front of the neck start to tense. These are some of the primary muscles involved in preventing forward head carriage, and they can get pretty weak after years of laptop life. So, keeping the position may take a bit of effort after a second or two. Don't do anything crazy; don't push too hard, but take a moment to notice those muscles and the powerful focus needed to keep your head stable.

This kind of focus is essential to repatterning, as you reorganize the tension patterns in your body back toward Healthy Neutral. For many of us, there will be a fair amount of work required to rebuild strength in the front of the neck. Take your time.

A healthy practice will integrate healthy skull position into postures.

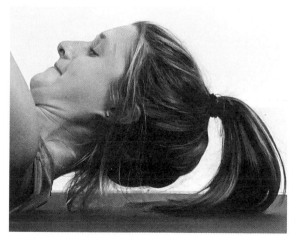

Look down your nose to really get the effect.

GOOD POSTURE CAN BE EXHAUSTING

We have all had that moment when, after hours at a device or in the car or at the computer, we notice we are sitting or standing with terrible posture. So we perk up, take a breath, get the spine and the shoulders and the skull in order, and resolve ourselves to sitting upright with our head high and our shoulders back and our eyes set clearly on a blue-sky future. And for a minute or so, it works. But after a while we get tired, and gravity kicks in, and everything starts to fall apart again. Pretty soon, we're back where we started, hunched over and glassy-eyed, wondering why we just can't seem to make good posture stick. We might think, hey, all of the internet articles say keeping my head over my shoulders uses less energy than forward head carriage, so what gives? Why is it so tiring to keep an upright position? Isn't that supposed to make things easier?

Yes and no. When the system is in balance, with the necessary strength to hold your head upright and your shoulders back, then upright posture comes easily. But if we haven't been holding upright posture for years, we may have to rebuild this strength to restore balance. The rebuild will take time and focus, but it's worth it.

3. Hypertonic Hip Flexors

Arguably the most important and detrimental effect sitting can have on your body occurs in and around your hips. Sitting in a chair puts your hips in flexion, where your thighs are about perpendicular to your torso. When your hips are in flexion, your hip flexors—a very important group that includes some of the largest muscles in your body, including your quadriceps and psoas muscles—can get *hypertonic,* which means they become overly rigid and gripped.

Basically, some very big, very important muscles adapt to fit the chair position. This is problematic for many reasons. For one, your hip flexors are responsible for lifting your legs forward when you walk (among a lot of other stuff). Every step you take will be influenced by tension in this group. Additionally, if your psoas major—which runs from your inner thigh to your lower back—becomes shortened, it can start to pull on the lower back. This may create low back tension, externally rotate your thighs (spin them outward from neutral), or both.

On the other hand, certain adaptations in the hip flexors will have the opposite effect. In the "sway back" position (which we will get to shortly), it is more likely that the hip flexors will be hypertonic—overactive—but in a lengthened position. In this case as well the psoas major in particular may still "pull" on the lower back, but within a different pattern. We will look at these differences and how to identify them in the section "Basic Postural Issues" below.

A healthy practice will include some kind of quad stretch or opening, and work toward returning hypertonic hip flexors to a healthy position.

4. Pelvic Tilt

When your hip flexors and quads get hypertonic, they can begin to alter the way your pelvis sits on top of your legs. Your rectus femoris—one of the four quadriceps and one of the largest muscles in the body—is attached to the front of your pelvis and can "tip" your pelvis forward when it's tight. Imagine a bowl with a string attached to one edge. If you pull that string downward, the bowl will begin to tip that way. This is a very simple example of pelvic tilt, a condition where a muscular imbalance—like shortened quads—can take the pelvis out of Healthy Neutral. When the front of the pelvis is pulled down like this, we call it anterior pelvic tilt (APT).

Similarly, sitting can create the opposite problem: posterior pelvic tilt. In this condition, the hamstrings in the back of the legs become short and hypertonic, pulling the back of the pelvis down. This can happen when we sit for a long time with the hips tucked under the spine.

The tilt of the pelvis is very important, in part because the pelvis is the foundation of the spine. If the pelvis is out of Healthy Neutral, the rest of the spine must compensate and may become accordingly misaligned. This will change the way you stand, walk, run, and practice yoga. Being able to identify and adjust the position of your pelvis, depending on the particular asana, is fundamental to a well-oriented practice.

A healthy yoga practice will emphasize a Healthy Neutral pelvic position.

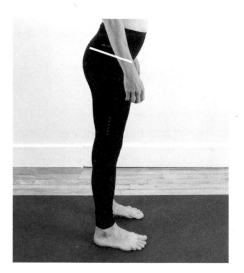

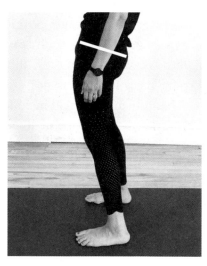

Anterior pelvic tilt.

Posterior pelvic tilt (with swayback).

5. Weak Glutes

Your glutes are the biggest muscles in your body. When healthy, they generate a whole lot of power. We like to sit on them because they're big and soft, which is a perk, but it's not the point. The main point of all that tissue is to generate the backward "drive" in your legs when you walk and run. (Also external rotation, but that's a whole different kettle.) They help stabilize your pelvis and—when they're healthy—can help relieve tension in your lower back and hips.

When you sit down, you sit primarily on your glutes (a.k.a. your butt, FYI). Prolonged pressure on these muscles can make them lose blood supply and tone. This can lead to something people sometimes called "gluteal amnesia," which frankly sounds like the worst spy movie ever made. Gluteal amnesia means that your butt muscles quite literally "forget" how to do their job. This is no good. If your glutes aren't well integrated into your walking stride, other muscles—like, say, your hip flexors or lower back muscles[30]—have to kick in more power than they're designed to provide. (It's like in a sci-fi movie when the aliens in the prosthetics damage some part of the human ship and the captain demands the crew "divert all power to thrusters!" to escape or whatever. Your body can do this; it can divert power from one area to another to get the job done, but then it's operating in some kind of emergency capacity and is probably in need of repair if it's going to be "fully operational."[31])

Like with every other maladaptation, there are more issues involved with weak and amnesiac glutes. Your glutes are important external rotators and pelvic stabilizers. We could write a whole book on just this one area of the body.[32]

A healthy yoga practice must have a substantial focus on activating and developing the glutes, and reintegrating them into functional movement.

---

[30] Your quadratus lumborum muscles, or QLs, particularly.

[31] By the way, I don't know if it's true, but I feel like that's got to be the first ever science-fiction spaceship combat reference in a yoga book. I'd like to thank the Academy.

[32] Which much smarter people than me have done. And let's be honest, if you're going to tell the world you're writing an entire book about butts, you'd better have some serious credentials. For example, check out Bret Contreras and Glen Cordoza, *Glute Lab: The Art and Science of Strength and Physique Training* (Las Vegas: Victory Belt, 2019).

6. Imbalanced Leg Strength

If your glutes aren't creating enough drive to send your legs back when you walk, then the odds are your hamstrings (which are also part of your "seat" when you're sitting down) aren't kicking on properly either. The hamstrings are part of a chain of action, the drive that propels the body forward. This drive is an important part of a healthy gait. I mean, it's more than "part"; it's like … literally half. The other half is the swing of the leg forward. There are lots of components to a healthy drive, but the chain of glutes-hamstrings-calves serves as its primary source of power. If that chain isn't healthy and strong, every step you take will require some kind of compensatory force to move. ("Divert power to thrusters" again.)

Remember when we said sitting down can make your quads hypertonic? That essentially means the front side of the legs—the chain that does the "swing" part of your gait, drawing your leg forward—can get too strong. *Too strong relative to what?* you might ask. Surely some people with freight-train quads have a healthy walking gait, right? Great question, hypothetical version of you. You're right, lots of people with freight-train quads walk perfectly well. When we say the quads can get "too strong" we mean too strong *relative to their antagonists*. Weird phrase, I know. Which means time for another insert.

AGONISTS VERSUS ANTAGONISTS

Muscle fibers are sort of dumb. They contract and relax, and that's mostly it. Any isolated muscle won't have a great amount of detailed control by itself. Movement becomes complex and exact not by the simple activation of muscles, but by the *coordination* of their activity. Your nervous system does the important work of organizing power; your muscles are simply generating said power.

When you lift your hand to pluck a fugitive eyelash from the face of a friend *(or enemy?)* your bicep contracts to bend your elbow. But that's not all that's happening. If only your bicep turned on, the bend of your elbow might lack control. In order to make the lift of your hand smooth and efficient, your triceps—on the opposite side of your arm—needs to turn on too, to counterbalance the bicep's action. So your nervous system coordinates the muscles on both sides of a joint and keeps the action smooth and stable.

In this action the bicep is the "agonist," it's the primary driver of the motion. The triceps is the "antagonist," it provides resistance to the agonist to keep the action under control. It's a beautiful system, when you think about it: two sides of a whole operating in a sort of cooperative resistance pattern, supporting each other through balanced opposition. Like the yin and the yang, working together by working against each other, your body follows the Rule of Three.

The "too" in "too strong" is relative to the system. It's like balancing a scale; there's no such thing as "too heavy" on a scale unless the other side is "too light." Unfortunately, when the weak hamstrings problem combines with the strong and tight quads problem, our walking patterns can become unbalanced. This can create a feedback loop where every step you take reinforces the imbalance in the system.

If this sounds bleak, take heart. You're the kind of person who reads yoga books, all the way to the hamstrings and quads section. You've got the commitment and information to start working on all this stuff. And it is work, for sure. But that's cool; what else are you going to do with your time: prop up an oppressive postmodern oligarchy? You're way too smart for that.

A healthy yoga practice should focus on balanced leg strength and tension patterns, especially the power of the hamstrings relative to the quads.

7. Inactive Core Muscles

When we say the "core," people some-times get different ideas, so we should clear this up before we go much far-ther. What exactly is a "core" on humans? Is a human being an apple? A planet? A thermonuclear reactor? Are we in danger of going critical or being stolen from an abandoned silo by rogue agents of a failed Soviet state? *Maybe?*

Some people say "core" in refer-ence to the entire axial body: pretty much everything except arms and legs. That's a nice definition, but it's a little broad for us. When we say "core" in this book, we mean the muscles of the abdomen and lower back, plus the pelvic floor and the diaphragm. For our purposes, it's not terribly productive to think about it in terms of individual muscles. Instead, think about your core as an integrated team of structures—muscle and con-nective tissue—that work together to coordinate movement and pressure throughout the torso.

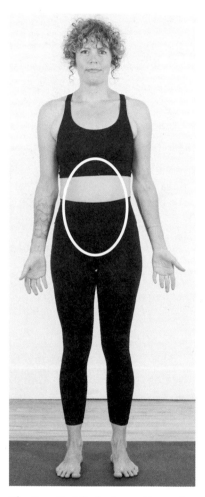

The "core" of the body, pretty much.

Crucially, your core helps stabilize your spine and distribute tension around and throughout the abdomen. It is a major portion of your pri-mary breathing structure. Belly breathing causes the core to expand and contract; chest breathing requires that the core remain somewhat stable; full torso breathing needs symmetrical and coordinated activation between the rib cage and the core.

When you walk or run—especially on uneven terrain[33]—your core is *constantly* reacting to balance your body as it shifts and bounces around. Meanwhile, you need air the whole time you're walking. So your core must help support your spine to keep you vertical, coordinate breathing structures to make sure you can take even, full breaths to meet your demand for oxygen, integrate the motion of leg and arm swinging, and protect many of your most vital organs. This is a lot of work. It requires a good degree of coordination and power. Luckily, it's what we've evolved to do and, normally, we do it quite well.

You are best suited to perform high-level athletic movements, like running or jiu-jitsu or heavy lifting, if your torso is stable in the process. (Weightlifters know this well: many of them even wear large core-stabilizing belts when doing particularly heavy lifts.[34]) You can see this in all sorts of athletic feats: watch Usain Bolt run or Alex Honnold climb or Serena Williams play a point or LeBron James do … anything. What you'll see is a relative capacity for twisting and bending the spine, but all in all things are more stable than not (particularly with sprinters and runners of any kind). High-level dancers are interesting to watch in this regard as well. Even when they throw themselves into wild positions, you will notice they display a tremendous ability to *limit* their motions as they generate inertia through movement.

And limiting this movement is no small feat. Your torso has weight, as do your arms and neck and head. For example, the average adult human head weighs about as much as a small-ish bowling ball. Let's sit with that for a second. You have the equivalent of a bowling ball perched atop your

---

[33] Which, in terms of human evolution, was pretty much the only kind of terrain. Not many Paleolithic *Homo sapiens sapiens* jogged around in their New Balances on level concrete.

[34] I should acknowledge here that some people love these belts and some people think they're counterproductive. Not going to take sides here, just stating that there isn't universal consensus on the value of this equipment. However, the point remains: The purpose of weightlifting belts is to help maintain core stability, particularly to protect your lower back.

neck, bobbing around, rotating, nodding, and headbanging to Alice in Chains. Take that in. Think of how much strength and support this structure demands whenever you're not lying down, particularly when you're in motion. It's a lot, friends. This strength is not exclusively provided by the structures of the neck; there's just not enough power there. Rather, it is integrated into and shared with the structures below (shoulders, arms, torso, etc.). Think now of the Josephine. Your neck is not just a neck; it's part of a comprehensive whole.

When you move around, your core has to adjust and reorient tension to make sure you don't fall over or collapse like a deflated bouncy house. However, when your butt is in a seat for most of the day, your core muscles don't need to react very much to keep you vertical. Your spine is already pretty stable (often because it's rounded forward and collapsed in on itself). What's more, you don't exactly have a huge oxygen demand when you're thumbing through Instagram, so your breathing gets shallow. This gets you in a feedback loop: your need for oxygen diminishes, so your core disengages, so your breathing gets shallower, so you move less, so your need for oxygen diminishes.

I think this is a good time to introduce an important concept: your posture and your breathing are connected. In fact, they're so connected that it's pretty safe to say your breathing and your posture are *the same thing*. That is, the way that you breathe *is* the way you hold yourself. This might sound weird, but just try something out real quick: take a big breath, nice and smooth all the way in and all the way out. I bet at some point during this breath—toward the top of the inhale, usually—your posture was more upright. (Or maybe you did that thing where you rearranged yourself to sit taller in preparation for taking a deep breath? Same difference.) Posture is not an abstract idea or a static position. How your postural muscles activate is how your breathing muscles activate because *they're the same exact muscles*.

See, the action of breathing is performed primarily by the contraction and relaxation of the muscles of your torso. Each and every one of these muscles is also a postural muscle in some way, because they influence the way you hold your spine, pelvis to skull. There is not an independent breathing structure and an independent postural structure; there is one structure performing two functions simultaneously.

A healthy yoga practice should integrate core engagement in coordination with full, dynamic breathing.

8. Lack of Rotation

Human bodies are made to rotate, especially when walking and running. A natural walking gait includes contralateral movement, which means when your right hip and leg move forward, your left chest and shoulder swing forward at the same time to balance the action. This is a remarkably efficient and elegant design. It makes us faster and more powerful while conserving energy. (There have actually been some pretty cool studies done on arm-swinging in human movement. Needless to say, if you tape someone's arms to their torso they are less balanced and use more metabolic energy with every stride. Also—and I'm just imagining here because I didn't personally participate in any of these studies—they look totally ridiculous.)

To keep our walking and running (and swimming and climbing and throwing, which generally involve rotation or contralateral motion as well) movements healthy, we need to allow for the transmission of energy to cross the body, from hip to opposite shoulder in particular. A particularly effective form of this is "open-chain" rotation, where certain extremities are not grounded against a point of contact; they're pretty much just hanging in space. Without the leverage provided by things like binds, the rotational muscles of the torso (things like the QLs and the lats and the transverse abs) must activate, balance, and cooperate in a well-integrated way.

The forward orientation of computers and televisions and car steering wheels and cell phones has another hidden consequence, beyond the more obvious forward head carriage and hunched shoulders. When sitting down, we don't often rotate. Our hips don't swing; neither do our arms and shoulders. (Because, you know, nothing much else is happening physically either.)

A healthy yoga practice should emphasize rotation and include open-chain action.

9. Forward Lean

Let's try something out. Stand up real quick. Now lift one leg up so you're standing on one foot. Hold it for a couple seconds. Now, feel your foot on the floor. Where is the weight landing through your foot? If you're like many others, when you stand on one leg (or both, but it's clearer when balancing) the weight of your body often carries forward over the toes.

Think about feet. (Weird line, Tarantino, but go with me.) Notably, think about where your ankle inserts into the foot. Where does that happen? The evolutionary design of the foot anchors the weight of the body in the posterior—rear—third of the foot. Give or take. Generally, when in Healthy Neutral, the weight of the body will be more over the heel than the forefoot. Pretty straightforward, right?

Now try standing on one foot again. Make sure you stay upright in your torso (don't pitch forward) and intentionally move the weight of your body back over your heel. What do you notice? Odds are, in this position your hamstrings and glutes have to fire more. You might even feel the abdominal muscles engage. The forward lean pattern often includes things like low back tension, sleepy glutes, and a disengaged abdominal wall.

There are additional factors involved in creating this forward shift,[35] but for now suffice to say it shows up a lot. In fact, one of the most common commands you'll hear in balancing poses during my class is "Ungrip your toes; anchor your heel." Not because this is a magic command, it's just almost always necessary. Most students I've worked with tend to shift forward and "grab" the floor with their toes when they balance on one leg.

A healthy yoga practice should include weight-bearing in the rear third of the foot during standing.

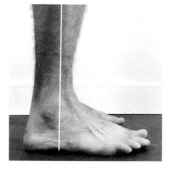

The line of the shin lands toward the back of the foot more than the front.

---

[35] I highly recommend Katy Bowman's books, particularly *Move Your DNA: Restore Your Health through Natural Movement* (Carlsborg, WA: Propriometrics Press, 2017), for more insight into the way things like shoes and flat floors mess up our feet and, by extension, pretty much everything else.

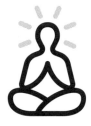

BASIC POSTURAL ISSUES

What's Going On and How to Spot It

Humans, like all organisms, are not standardized. Evolution requires and imposes variation in all living things, so it is impossible to create rules that fit perfectly with every individual and type of person. We're just too interesting to be contained that way.

That being said, there are places where we can reach a general understanding about the major patterns in life. Stuff like: you probably shouldn't try to make your cat a vegan, and a semi-consistent bedtime will probably improve your daily mood. Might not be the case for everyone, but it's helpful to know the basic trends.

In terms of human postural maladaptive patterns, we'll address four major ones: lordosis, kyphosis, sway back, and flat back. Each of these patterns has a unique set of concerns. We will touch on the major points of each and how they tend to influence yoga poses, and provide possible corrections. Before we continue, sign the waiver. This is not medical advice.

Lordosis

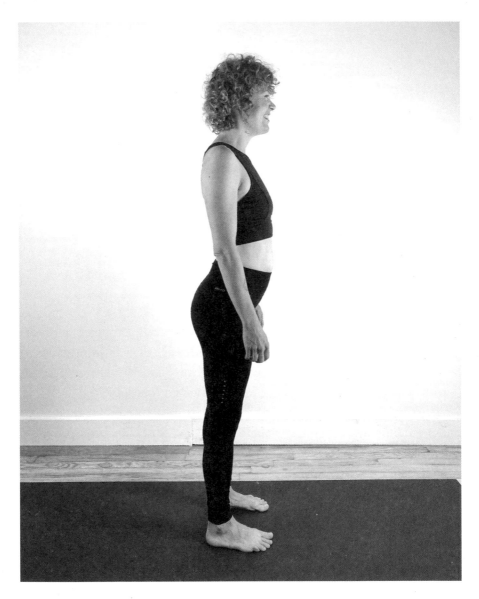

So named for the spinal curves in the lower back and neck, this pattern includes:

- anterior pelvic tilt
- forward thrust of the ribs
- hyperextension in the neck and lower back

The tilt of the pelvis will likely mean the hamstrings are pulled long and the lower belly has pushed forward. The human might have shortened the hip flexors in this position as well. Developing strength in the core, glutes, and the front of the neck may help pattern toward neutral.

This body pattern "hides" in yoga poses very well, particularly when a practice emphasizes back bends, since the student has a sort of preexisting back bend—in which the lordotic curve puts the lumbar spine into near-constant hyperextension—that can be exploited to allow greater depth in back-bending postures. However, when the spine is placed into flexion, like in Pyramid or Wild Child, it's quite common to discover humans with lordosis are unable to effectively round their spines. Instead, the tendency is for the spine to remain flat as a board from the sacrum all the way to the mid-thoracic region.

When working with this body pattern, we should usually explore: abdominal strength, to reintegrate the connection between the ribs and pelvis on the front side; upper back strength, to encourage the upper back to reintegrate and stabilize toward neutral; and hamstring engagement, to start to balance against anterior pelvic tilt.

Kyphosis

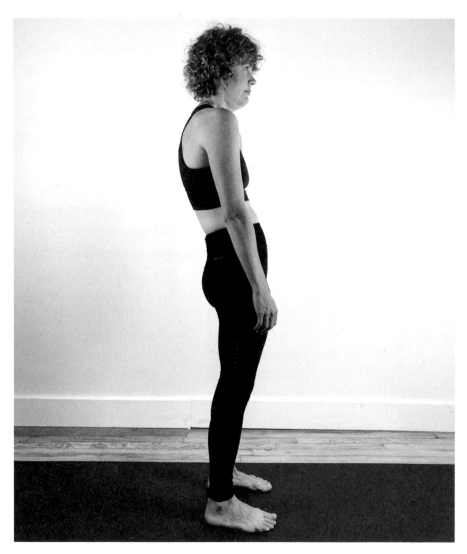

Here the upper spine shifts back and the shoulders shift forward, which creates a hunch in the upper back. Concurrently, the skull shifts forward to balance the whole system.

Common signs and symptoms are:

* anterior pelvic tilt
* forward head carriage
* shoulder hunch
* hyperextended knees

In kyphosis a collapse in the backward lean of the upper back is often complimented by a collapse in the lumbar spine and anterior pelvic tilt. Back bending poses will occasionally be more accessible to a person with kyphosis, while flexion in the lumbar spine will likely be a real challenge.

Students with kyphosis will most likely benefit from heart-opening positions that simultaneously strengthen and stabilize the upper back. Think Cobra and Crocodile particularly. Core strength and healthy mobility in the lower back—as in Wild Child or Pyramid—will also be beneficial.

ON CHANGING EXPECTATIONS

Students sometimes get annoyed or frustrated with practices that challenge their existing patterns. If you're doing something to create fundamental change, it will always be more difficult than following existing routines. Basically, if something is easy for you, it's probably not going to modify your patterns.

Lordosis and kyphosis are, to varying degrees, quite common among the general population of modern humans. Some people may have long-term yoga practices that not only allow for but reinforce their existing patterns. Some may have developed "deep" or "advanced" poses that take advantage of their existing patterns, reinforcing them in the process. The work is to mindfully adjust our perspective on what the ultimate aim of the practice is; instead of chasing poses, shift patterns.

Sway Back

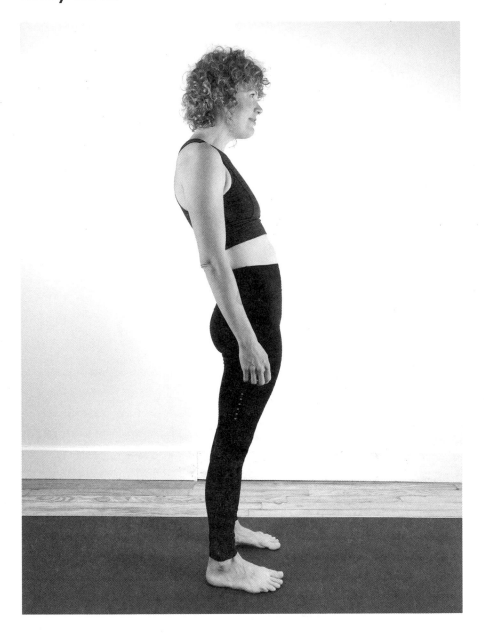

Here the whole body "bows" forward as the hips shift forward beyond the line of gravity. You could encompass it fairly well (though not completely) by just saying, "the front body gets loose and the back body gets tight."

- posterior pelvic tilt
- forward head carriage
- hyperextended knees

In an attempt to balance out this bowing action, the head pushes forward of the shoulders. So once again we have forward head carriage. However, forward head carriage may not be as apparent here as in kyphosis, because the backward "lean" of the torso makes the neck stand upright in relation. The relative angle of the neck and rib cage is one of forward head carriage, but the cervical spine is often somewhat neutral to the line of gravity.

A good way to investigate this idea is to take a picture and present it from two different angles. Check it out. In picture 1, I'm standing in the "swayback" pattern. You can see that the position of my skull is pretty vertical, right? So you might decide that I don't have forward head carriage. From one perspective, you'd be right. However, note the angle between my rib cage and neck.

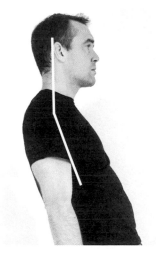

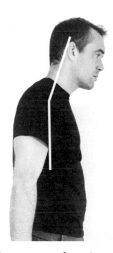

Picture 1.

Picture 2: just a rotated version of picture 1.

Now look at picture 2. Here's the trick: picture 2 is the same as picture 1. It's just been rotated so my rib cage is fairly vertical, about where it would be in Healthy Neutral. Now we can see that the skull is forward of the shoulders. If we simply look at someone with their head upright and determine they don't have forward head carriage, we might be missing some important information. Namely, what is the relationship of the skull with the rest of the spine? It's important to keep in mind that Healthy Neutral is not simply about the line of gravity, but also about the relative orientation of different parts of the body.

In yoga poses, particularly balancing poses, people with this pattern will often maintain the forward bow in their bodies. Look to reset the vertical line of hips-over-ankles, in particular. This will often be quite challenging, and might even make some students fall over a couple of times. Keep at it; it will help reintegrate core strength and return to Healthy Neutral.

Flat Back

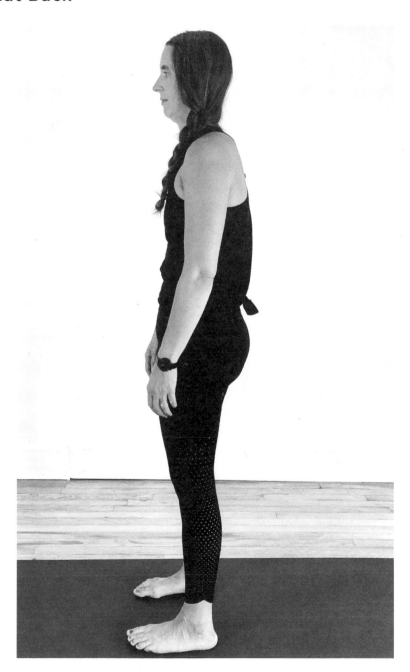

Here the pelvis is "tucked" into a posterior tilt, flattening the lower back.

- posterior pelvic tilt
- flat mid- and lower back
- externally rotated femurs (often)
- hamstrings short and tight

In this pattern the posterior chain is quite strong, perhaps even locked up, holding the human upright strongly but often limiting range of motion. Moving the spine—particularly into flexion—can be a struggle for people with this pattern. The hamstrings are often "locked" tightly here. It's the pattern of many people who cannot touch their toes. You may notice limitations in the posterior chain elsewhere in the ankles, calves, and back of the neck.

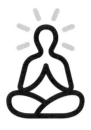

EFFICIENCY MACHINES

I f all of this seems like a lot, I get it. It is. And there's a lot more; these are just the major concerns, as far as I can tell. But we should integrate this kind of information into the conversation about a healthy yoga practice, at least when we're talking about the physical practice, because body patterns do not magically disappear when we enter a yoga room. Warrior 1 does not exist outside of your patterns; it moves within them. If we are going to put together a posture—any posture at all—with intelligence, we need to take body patterns into account.

Remember, your body is an efficiency machine. It wants to do stuff—especially challenging stuff like yoga poses—with as little energy as possible. That's what evolution designed our bodies to do: use any and all shortcuts available, and our bodies learned their lesson well. The upshot is, when your body is trying to maintain a posture, it's going to "choose" the patterns it already has, things that are already strong.

For example, if I'm doing Chair Pose, my body is likely going to "want" to do a version where my core is disengaged, and my lower back collapses, and my skull moves forward of the shoulders, and the back of my neck grips, and the weight of my body is in my toes. If those are my patterns, that's what my body wants to use. In terms of energy, making new patterns is expensive. It's cheapest to just use (and, by extension, reinforce) what's already there.

To practice yoga postures however they "come naturally" is not always an optimal method of practice. At least not by itself, though I wish it were. I wish that our daily routines matched our evolutionary design. I wish we all had balanced patterns and were nicely aligned with Healthy Neutral—which I believe is our birthright—but a lot of us don't have that stuff these days. For many people in the modern world, there are deeply ingrained maladaptive patterns in their bodies.

Another way to look at it is to consider preventative medicine versus curative medicine. Yoga gets a lot of press as a preventative method; it keeps you healthy so you don't have issues later. And this is totally true. But anyone who's gone to a yoga class to get over a bad day at the office also knows that yoga has curative elements. It *fixes* stuff. The work of the practice is in part the work of balancing out the burdens modernity foists on us every day.

THIS IS WATER

It's important we take a second to acknowledge that this lifelong sitting and body-pattern problem is not any individual person's fault. My genuine hope is that we can explore these challenges with an absence of judgment. We all start where we are. The work is the work; it is not a sign of failure or lack.

This all started before we were truly in control of our lives. By the time we had agency, many of us were so deeply patterned by sitting that we probably started to seek it out. And that might be where you are right now: sitting in a chair or on the couch might feel like the most comfortable, natural thing you could do with your time. And honestly, part of that feeling is true; show me a primate who doesn't enjoy a plush microsuede sectional and I'll show you an orangutan that knows how to lie.

It's not your fault if you like chairs. I like chairs too. This is simply the water that we swim in. Our context and our background are not personal flaws. Just like it's not a teenager's fault he loves his cell phone; those things are cripplingly addictive by design, and he got it when he was seven years old. How was he supposed to resist? Our culture trains us to do things that aren't good for us, and it's been refining this process for thousands of years. You didn't create your environment; you came into it. It is your karma. Which is another way of saying, it's what we work with.

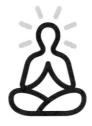

DIRTY ROTTEN CHEATERS

t doesn't really matter how much good information someone has if they're pushed too hard. If a posture is too complex or sends them to their physical edge, a student is probably going to abandon repatterning and immediately revert to habit. We only have so much energy to contribute at any given moment.

For example, one time David Hasselhoff came into the Banana Republic where I was working in Santa Monica, like 15 years ago,[36] and he was all worked up because he needed white clothes for Puff Daddy's White Party, where you're only allowed to wear pure white and nothing else, and he was in a huge hurry because he was running behind, and the party was on a boat, and the boat would in fact leave the dock at some point, so being "fashionably late" meant being left on dry land while Puff and Mace and Tobey Maguire threw their hands skyward and swayed to island beats as Pacific breezes ruffled their linen button-ups, and, well, for Mr. Hasselhoff such an absence would, I imagine, be a personal and possibly even a professional calamity. So anyway, the problem was that Banana Republic didn't really *do* white that year, because they were really leaning into eggshell and tan and canvas and beige, and Mr. Hasselhoff was getting a bit flush in the face as he smacked hangers in frustration. And, well, I was trying to help.

---

[36] This really happened.

If the situation had been less urgent, I might have been able to take a breath and regretfully concede we had nothing—though Zara probably did—and maybe also remark to David that I considered his capacity for macho-schlock acting to be its own kind of art, a skill that is frankly underappreciated in the realm of television performance. But I didn't. I had one task, and it was quite pressing—Puff awaited—so I lost focus on the details: how I could really help and maybe even give someone a compliment. And so I spent the whole ten minutes scampering around in a craze trying to find the whitest chinos in the building with little success. By the time Mr. Hasselhoff left, empty-handed, I was a nervous wreck and needed to take lunch early. I never did find out if he made the boat.

In the rush of a challenging experience, I was not able to slow down and act in the way I would have liked. We have all felt something similar, something challenging happened one day, and instead of taking a moment to mindfully address the details, we acted on habit and impulse. Right?

I think yoga students and teachers should reflect: what is the point of complex or "advanced" poses? They undoubtedly impose a greater need for focus and concentration. In fact, that is often their explicit value. But this inherently means students have less focus for work besides just trying to get in the pose at all. Are these forms, these poses, providing a benefit that outweighs their potential to reinforce habit?

I'm not trying to push any particular answer. How you choose to approach the practice depends on your personal goals. I just think sometimes yoga teachers and students can get a little cavalier about chasing super-duper poses because they're fun and impressive and a gold mine for social media. If you're a dancer or a gymnast or something, and you're already strong and flexible and physically balanced in Healthy Neutral, you may not need the extra focus required for repatterning. I personally love a bunch of advanced poses, but I don't teach them to people who are still in the repatterning stages of their practice.

Because even if a student *can* do a pose, it may not serve them to do so. I can't tell you how many "bendy" students I have seen recruit and reinforce their habits just to achieve things like deep back bends and complex binds. Or how many handstanders I have watched sink into their lower backs and grip their necks simply to stay inverted. It's not that recruiting these old patterns will wreck your body in thirty seconds flat, but it probably won't help the long-term work of balancing your body's systems.

When it comes to posture selection, we must consider our overall goals. In terms of repatterning, an effective posture is not only manageable, it actively orients the practice toward Healthy Neutral. This central work must be emphasized, supported, and reinforced not just philosophically but physically. In time, once we have repatterned a bit toward Healthy Neutral, we can increase the challenge in the practice. But adding undue challenge to the system before we have the fundamentals down risks reinforcing maladaptive patterns.

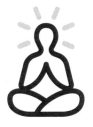

RECAP

Using these central ideas—evolutionary design, Healthy Neutral, and repatterning—we can build an intentional yoga practice. Our mission is to practice with respect for basic components and imperatives of human evolution, as best we understand them, in order to bring the body back toward balance and integration.

Before we dive back down into the postures and assemble the Foundations of Repatterning, let's recap the physical stuff from part one.

For all-level students in the modern world, a healthy yoga practice should:

- open the front of the chest while simultaneously strengthening the upper back to restore healthy balance around the rib cage and shoulders

- integrate healthy skull position into postures, including a release of hyperextension in the neck

- include some kind of quad stretch or opening, and work toward releasing and strengthening tight hip flexors

- emphasize neutral pelvic position

- focus on developing and reintegrating the glutes into movement

- focus on balanced leg strength and tension patterns, including especially the power of the hamstrings
- integrate core engagement in coordination with dynamic breathing
- emphasize rotation
- emphasize weight-bearing in the rear half of the foot

We want these benefits of the practice to show up in two ways: posture selection and teaching cues. Basically, we want to select poses that emphasize these benefits, and we want to teach the poses we select in a way that maximizes their efficacy.

OK. Thanks for sticking with me through all that. I think you'll find it beneficial as you approach your own yoga practice. Now let's get going with the Foundations of Repatterning.

PRACTICE:
THE FOUNDATIONS
OF REPATTERNING
(A.K.A. "FOUNDATIONS")

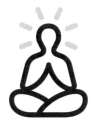

ABOUT THE SEQUENCE

The Foundation of Repatterning is a yoga practice designed from the ground up to meet the needs of human beings in the modern world. It draws its primary yoga influence from Bikram and Anusara[37] while integrating some concepts from Ashtanga, YogaHour, and Yin. It is the result of synthesis, trial and error, exploration, conversation, and a continued willingness to throw away anything that didn't work.

We want this practice to be:

All levels: Accessible to beginners and challenging for "advanced" students. Novices should be able to safely do the poses without injuring themselves or unconsciously cheating all over the place. This is easier said than done. Many "standard" yoga poses are exceedingly difficult to teach to a group of beginners without reinforcing maladaptive patterns. For example, many people can cross one leg in Half Lotus, but very few can safely and effectively sit in the pose without putting stress on their knee or rounding their spine or collapsing their ankle or, you know, all kinds of stuff.

Over time, we've done our best to find the most accessible poses while challenging experienced students, and have retaining a wide variety of

---

[37] It's purely coincidence that both of these methods achieved wild success by innovating on established practices, became objects of maniacal devotion during their height, and suffered devastating scandals involving their "guru" figures. Go figure.

movements in the practice. It wasn't easy; we cut many beloved postures from the sequence because we just couldn't figure out how to teach them in a way that avoided rampant cheating and took less than fifty-three hours.

Functional: Help develop functional mobility and strength. Remember, *the poses are not the point.* They're the practice, the tool we use to get something else. In Foundations, one major way we measure success is by the ability of our students to do, you know, normal stuff. We don't care if you can touch your toes to your eyebrows (OK, that's a little bit of a lie. Scorpion looks pretty awesome. But we're not going for that, here). We *do* care if you can walk for ninety minutes without pain, or help your cousin move into a split-level, or toss an office-size printer down a fire escape. You know: normal stuff.

Ritualized: In a yoga class, the more brain power we have to use on figuring out the basic format of the next pose, the less brain power we have on *organizing* that pose in terms of alignment. If we repeat a sequence regularly, we can get over the basics of "left foot forward, arms out, back heel down" and start to engage in the detailed work of repatterning. Ritualized sequences also have the benefit of connecting students as a group. People are drawn together by developing a common skill set, and ritual movement performs this function very well.

Good for groups: One of the vital benefits of yoga is social. While many students have developed a home practice (which is wonderful) most still use studios and group classes as their primary mode of practice. There is tremendous value in doing something with other human beings, particularly when we involve our bodies. Movement in unison draws people together. In Foundations we aspire to create a practice that may be taught generally, where the teacher does not need to specifically instruct each individual student. This style is common in the yoga world. However, teaching a diverse group of students, beginner to advanced, without leading a large portion of the group to reinforce habits? That's not easy. Human bodies are unique. Their needs are unique. Even the most experienced teacher must pay close attention to provide value, structure, and safety to groups larger than, I don't know, three people.

The posture selection for Foundations is explicitly oriented to meet this challenge. How can we provide the most value to the broadest spectrum of humans (within a reasonable time frame)? As such, we have worked to avoid: poses that are easily misunderstood; poses whose misalignments are particularly subtle and require direct personal attention from the teacher; poses that become significantly easier as your practice progresses. In Foundations we aim to create easy points of entry for all poses, provide a natural path to increased challenge, and keep the whole group safe with simple instruction.

Enjoyable: We can go around and around trying to make the practice as functional and helpful as possible (and we will), but every now and then we need to stop and remind ourselves: look, this can't just be medicine; you gotta toss some sugar on that cough syrup. Not many people—me, especially—want to make a yoga routine out of seventy-five- or ninety-minute group PT sessions. That's not exactly … fun. Life is short. Finding the shared space between "helpful" and "joyful" is important.

Relevant: Our practice should honestly engage the needs of twenty-first-century students, according to their particular and historically unique physical needs.

The hope with this practice is to create a ritual that will help students create balance in their bodies and mitigate maladaptive patterns. We should be clear: the goal is not always to *eliminate* maladaptive patterns. For most students—who have to continue their routines at work and home and can't just rebuild their entire lives from the ground up—the best approach helps unclench habitual patterns a bit, and gives them access to more diverse, healthier movement potential.

On Saints and Animals

During the early years of my practice, I developed a pretty intense obsession with enlightenment. In my entire life I had not encountered an idea so appealing, this concept that I might somehow—through practice—become a sage or even a Buddha. I imagined conquering significant emotional suffering and transcending attachment, shedding my earthly skin to reveal a better, higher version of myself. In these imaginings of my future incarnation, I was sometimes slightly bioluminescent.[38]

Deep down, what I was really interested in that whole time was becoming a different form of human being. The idea of universal suffering rang true to me. I was in pain and saw other humans in pain wherever I looked. (The news didn't help.) I began to believe that mankind needed a sort of level-up, an "evolutionary leap" beyond ourselves into the next stage of development or progress.[39] Yoga and meditation were pathways to a new Eden, filled with the new angels.

A common metaphor for this kind of thinking is the caterpillar-butterfly dichotomy, in which a lesser being (caterpillar) enters into a transformative stage (chrysalis) and in time becomes a higher being (butterfly). While this is an appealing idea, it's got some serious flaws with regard to actual life in the world. Not the least of which is how demeaning it is to caterpillars. Who says a caterpillar is a lesser form of a butterfly? Sure, the aim of the natural life cycle of a caterpillar is to become a butterfly, but the aim of the natural life cycle of a butterfly is to *make caterpillars.* So ... who made the call that one of them is better than the other?

---

[38] To be clear, I'm not knocking the idea of enlightenment. What I'm saying is my personal concept of enlightenment was ill-formed. Presently, I'm pretty neutral on the idea. It sounds great, but I'm not currently formatting my daily life around it.

[39] Somewhat relevant: I have met a couple of people in the fitness world who promote the idea that human bodies are at a "mid-stage" in evolution, that they're not "done" evolving yet. The theory is that humans develop pain as they age, and their bodies start to fall apart, because somewhere in our evolutionary history we lost the survival pressure to evolve "better" bodies. Our brains got good at keeping us alive before our bodies could finish evolving. I hate this idea. Mainly I hate it because it's nihilistic and defeatist. What is the value in telling people their bodies are not fully formed? And also, that's not really how evolution works. Evolution does not have a trajectory; it is an ongoing, survival-based relationship with current conditions. There's no plan. There are no "middle stages." Every point on the line of evolution is its apex. You are—right now, right here—the very best evolution could do. There is no other form of human being that we failed to reach. You're not halfway done; you're here.

The butterfly metaphor celebrates growth and change, which is good, but within it is the idea that human beings have the capacity, or even the responsibility, to become non-human beings … or post-human beings … or Übermensch … it's all a little hazy. The implication is that we are born in a lower form and our charge in life is to become a higher form through diligence and practice. Through this process a human becomes something like a saint, so we will call this idea the Saintly Model.

The Saintly Model is popular—I believe it dominates mainstream American culture—but it's not an established truth or anything. There are countless anecdotes regarding the spiritual transformation of human beings into something better, though there aren't many confirmed cases.[40] The Dalai Lama is an amazing person, sure, but he's not a different species or anything. He's not bioluminescent; he's just super-duper kind.

A contrary concept might be something we'll call the Animal Model, which basically means that you—as a piece of nature—are already fully formed. There is no "higher" version of you, though you can certainly refine and reshape yourself according to ideals and practices you choose to follow. In this model, "saint" is not an alternative state of being but rather a title for a very accomplished, but also very human, human being. The animal is still the animal. The Dalai Lama still chews with his mouth bones and gets boogers and sleeps.

The central idea of the Animal Model is that *human beings do not become non-human beings*. As I said in the beginning, a human being may be defined in all sorts of ways. Regardless of how you define "human," the point is you are already one and won't become anything else within this lifetime. This approach is maybe a little less romantic than the Saintly Model, since it means you can't really transcend your basic nature. However, the Animal Model is far from hopeless. Like every other form of life on this planet, human beings are brilliant creatures. We have the capacity for remarkable athleticism, unparalleled problem solving, and social

---

[40] No, Facebook posts about some dude who sat in deep meditation under a tree without food or water for like seventy years and is still somehow alive and *scientists are baffled* do not count as "confirmed cases."

coordination of the highest order, among other talents. We don't have to transform into amazing things; we are amazing things.

Of course, it's sometimes hard to see this amazingness. Being human is often stressful and fraught. It can be difficult to cultivate a sense of harmony and flow within our lives. Part of this has to do with time and place. There is undeniably some sort of imbalance between human beings and the environments we have created for ourselves. Civilization has brought forth amazing wonders, but as we've discussed (extensively; oh, my god, I'm so sorry) it's also sort of … off. We don't exactly fit into the spaces we have built for ourselves. It's understandable that, within a context where we may feel out of place, we conjure fantasies about becoming different things entirely. This is unfortunate, in part because if we tell ourselves that we *should* fit neatly into modern life but are fundamentally *incapable* of doing so, we might get the bad idea that we're some kind of grand human failure.

Which, to be very clear, we—you, I, all of us—are not. Our world has some serious issues we should all take responsibility for, but if you feel out of whack with your environment and the modern way of life, that's not your fault. We were built for a different world, and that world is now almost entirely gone.

To be clear, I'm not an advocate for the noble savage concept. I don't believe humans were once perfected beings that held the secrets of the universe in their hearts and, I don't know, caught birds on their fingertips like Cinderella. Nor do I believe that humans once lived in painless bliss, or that fear and sadness were alien to our prehistoric ancestors. It's not like that. Lions kill their prey by biting their necks. Chimpanzees sometimes carry out brutal territorial conflicts. Humans have a long history—and prehistory—of murdering each other. Life is wild. And we are life. This isn't an attempt to excuse violence or bad behavior; it's just to say our condition has its benefits and its challenges. One of those challenges is maintaining our balance in the world as it is.

Animals in captivity—trapped within environments that are out of sync with their evolutionary design—often develop behavioral signs of chronic stress, PTSD, and other mental illnesses. Recall how tigers pace back and forth in their cages, which is an indication they are chronically anxious.

Imagine if one day a pacing tiger did some honest self-study and discovered she is filled with emotional stress. This makes the tiger very sad. She wants to get better. So she decides she is going to work and work and work to fix the problem. Her goal is to work so hard that one day she will turn into a unicorn, because everybody has heard that unicorns don't have any stress.[41]

This is obviously absurd. The problem isn't that tigers should be unicorns and this one is not. The problem is she's in an environment that doesn't suit her. So the best solution is not transmute the stress of being a caged tiger. The best solution is get out of the cage. Human beings are sort of like this. We have constructed an elaborate, pervasive cage for ourselves. (It's actually an embedded hierarchy of interwoven cages.[42]) Yoga is not the work of gilding the cage; it is the work of freedom.

In Foundations we operate from the belief that a human being—any human being anywhere—is a marvelous thing. There is within each of us an ancient wisdom, a brilliant history written deeply into our genes. That we were born at all is a miracle beyond comprehension. We are challenged by our environment, it's true, but that is not a mandate to change our fundamental nature.[43] Our mandate is to understand ourselves more deeply and hold strongly to the marvelous humanity that is our birthright.

There is no escaping civilization (which would be silly to try anyway, because, I mean, where else are you going to find vegan gelato and true-crime podcasts?), but there is still opportunity to discover a greater sense of physical and psychological freedom. We can open for ourselves a space to stand up for what matters in life, to defy structures that demand we

---

[41] This is actually a common misconception. Unicorns are perfectionists, which can make unpredictable situations almost unbearable. This is part of the reason you don't see them often; they find it impossible to relax in public. Also, they're imaginary.

[42] These embedded cages include (in no particular order) patriarchy, white supremacy, late-stage capitalism, individualism, and convenience, to name a few.

[43] Encouraging you to change your fundamental nature is a rhetorical tool of capitalism, BTW ... *Feel oppressed by your office? Try these (proprietary) self-transformation techniques! Manage/repress negative emotion! Ignore the effects of meaningless oppressive environments! Increase your productivity 37 percent! For retirement savings!*

become anything other than what we are, and to work to restore a more humane—and human—way of life. As we do this, keep in mind some of the things that help human beings thrive: social groups, physical contact, routine, present awareness, and varied physical movement. Where can we find such things? Well, for starters, we can find them in yoga classes.

I sincerely believe this discussion is important for yoga students and teachers both. You don't have to agree with me, but I'd encourage you to investigate your approach to your practice. Do you choose the Saintly Model or the Animal Model? Are we trying to be higher-order humans or simply human? You can choose what you like. But now you know where I stand, you hopefully have a better sense of the ideas that formed Foundations.

Building Foundations

The aim of this book isn't to be a practice guide, in a strict sense. It is, at its heart, an investigation of ideas. We're going to use the postures as a vehicle for exploration, like the Apollo spacecraft or my Aunt Edith's Saab that one time she got us all lost in the Boston suburbs in 1988. When we're done unpacking Foundations, we will have thoroughly covered the essential tenets of the practice and the ways they inform various body positions.

We will describe the physical shapes, refine them with an eye for common issues, and then see if we can't use the practice to facilitate a sort of experiential learning. The basic format will be setup, entrance, assessment, breathing, options, goals.[44] Some poses will also include an Exit section, where that applies.

Setup: In this stage we'll go over the ways you prepare the body for the pose, without actually getting into it yet. This stage is vital. Sometimes it will have many steps. The point of setup is to make sure you're approaching the pose in a way that minimizes the tendency to "cheat." It preemptively addresses common misalignments. Think of it as a kind of preventative medicine: if we can anticipate common issues, we can help keep them from fully establishing themselves and messing up our poses.

---

[44] Except for the breathing exercises.

Entrance: This is the process for actually getting into the pose itself, usually coupled with a prescribed breathing pattern. The last few steps of entering a pose are often essential to the process. If it all falls apart here, we might as well reset and start over. I like to think about it like driving a car; if you discover there is something wrong with your vehicle, you don't try to fix it while you're in motion. Instead, you pull over, turn the engine off, fix the problem, then start driving again. Yoga poses can be sort of like that. It is a lot harder to fix them once they're in motion.[45]

Assessment: Here you're actually in the pose, so we're feeling it out, exploring the experience, and making available adjustments. Assessment is a good time to notice our tendencies, make minor fixes, and investigate the central concepts at play in the posture.

Breathing: In breathing we will discuss the orientation and value of the breath in the pose. We will also introduce some central concepts like, "every breath is a rep" and "Investigative Breathing." Sometimes breathing will involve in-depth descriptions and investigations. Sometimes it will be as simple as "breathe naturally."

Options: Here we will explore alternative ways to approach the postures. Some alternatives will increase the difficulty of the poses. Others will make them easier. I'll also provide some guidance on ways to use props during poses. If you're having trouble setting up a pose in a healthy, manageable way, check the options section. Likewise, if you feel well established in a pose and want to explore some more challenging alternatives, there might be something in this section for you as well.

Goals: For each posture we will include a little description of what the pose is trying to achieve and how it fits into the sequence as a whole. In Foundations, our central pursuit is to help you establish and maintain Healthy Neutral. For many students this takes more strength work. For others it will require more mobility work. It will likely be some sort of combination for you. Feel it out. Just know that our goal is not "get super-bendy" or "get super-strong." Our goal is a stable, balanced system.

---

[45] "Motion" in this context really just means we've fully entered the pose.

As we explore the practice, you'll also notice occasional notes regarding the Josephine and the Rule of Three. These will highlight opportunities for understanding where we might notice interconnectedness and the role of opposites in practice.

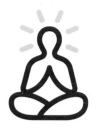

THE PRACTICES

Breathing

Pulling Down the Heavens

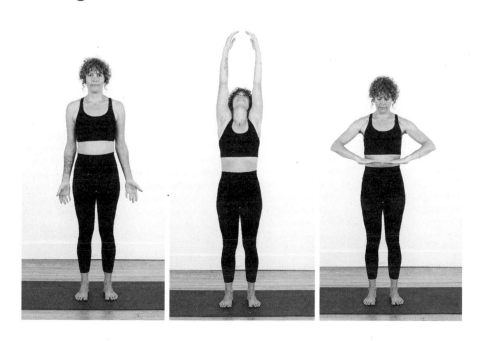

We begin with a breathing exercise we stole wholesale from Qigong, a traditional Chinese practice that combines breath and movement in a manner similar to some yoga practices. We use Pulling Down the Heavens as a form of intentional grounding, a way to set the mind and body into a place of comfortable focus for the class.

All you do is set your feet hip width apart and put a little bend in your knees. Be nice and relaxed to start.

Inhale slowly through the nose and sweep your arms overhead in a smooth, wide, slow circle. Look up to your thumbs and let your fingertips al-l-lmost touch.

Exhale through your mouth in a long sigh. Keeping your fingertips close to one another, smoothly bring your hands down through the midline of the body.

Do this (at least) three times.

Qi Gong teachers often describe this practice like you're gathering a ball of energy overhead and gently moving it down the front of the body—past the face, heart, and hips—to the ground beneath you.

Remember, the goal here is to center you in your body and in your practice. We're not yet in the weeds of anatomical neutral or alignment or whatever; we're simply acknowledging the breath and the body as we begin.

Reverse Anatomical Breathing

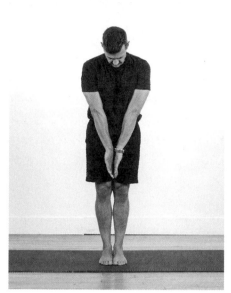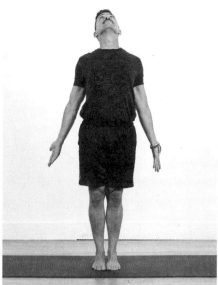

You may have encountered Anatomical Breathing before in yoga class. It's a classic. It works with what we might call our "natural" breathing patterns. That is; inhales moving up, exhales moving down; inhales opening the chest, exhales dropping the ribs; inhales back-bending, exhales rounding forward, etc. A standard Cat-Cow does the same thing with its inhale-up, exhale-down structure.

We just took this standard process and reversed it. (Total Kanye move, right?) It goes like this:

Inhale through your nose as you tuck your chin to look down, and bring the backs of the hands together in front of you.

Pause.

Exhale through your mouth, look up, open your chest, and turn your palms out.

That's it. You can let a little sway of the body in if you like, back and forth.

When we do it this way, the breathing will likely feel less "intuitive" or "natural" than in the normal format. We hear that a lot from students. We also hear occasionally that they don't "like" it as much as the original format. This is sort of the point.

Reverse Anatomical Breathing is an exercise in intentional resistance. We are engaging the tension that arrives when we behave in nonhabitual patterns. That you don't intuitively "want" to move this way is part of the reason we do it. From the beginning of the class, we are planting the concept that repatterning requires countermeasures, actions *against* our habits.

And this isn't merely about your mental perspective; it is profoundly physical as well. In fact, through this breathing pattern, we introduce some concepts vital to Foundations:

1. Moving inhales into the back body.

2. Intentionally activating core strength on both sides of the breath cycle.

3. "Flipping" an established practice—turning it on its head, you might say—to explore the power of opposition.

RULE OF THREE:
TRADITION VERSUS EXPERIMENTATION

Yoga is the product of experimentation. Human beings with remarkable curiosity, insight, and patience developed the practices through trial and error, feeling out what worked and what did not. When we hold to tradition, we honor this previous work, partly in the faith that these experiments were effective.

Tradition is an astonishingly efficient way to transmit information through generations. For example, if I wanted to learn how to make sourdough bread I could either invent sourdough bread from scratch by myself (never happening) or I could talk to a baker and learn the sourdough tradition (anybody got a good starter lying around?) Before reading and writing came along, tradition was our primary way of sharing important knowledge. To maintain a tradition you have to be careful to avoid unnecessary change. If something works, don't mess with it. Just trust the process, you know?

But what happens when you decide you want to make sourdough that's *better* than the recipe from Tartine?[46] (Why? I don't know; maybe palates have changed, or you're newly gluten-free.) In that case, you would start to experiment. One way to perform an experiment is to mess with tradition. Start with the recipe, switch things up, perform some actions backward, and see what happens.

And through this sort of experimentation, we learn more about tradition. We figure out what works and why it's there. What's truly essential and what can be modified or discarded completely. What's fluffy and spongy and delightful and what's burnt toast.

Experimentation and tradition inform, resist, and change one another. Because they are opposites, their interaction is creative. Reverse Anatomical Breathing is a very simple example of this creative interaction. Something traditional is experimented with (reversed, in this case) to create something different.[47] This is the Rule of Three in action.

---

[46] Tall order. Good luck.

[47] If you're interested, the story here is actually one step more involved than this. The "reversal" of the breath was something I first came across in Katonah Yoga, but in this case it was in Cat-Cow breathing. That principle was then applied to our practice. So again we see the dynamic; experimentation on the Cat-Cow breathing tradition created a new tradition (Katonah variation) which informed experimentation on another tradition (Anatomical Breathing) to create RAB, which is now its own sort of tradition.

Opening Sequence

Every morning when my dog wakes up, he sighs, rolls on his back, and electrocutes himself in slow motion. At least that's what it looks like. He stretches out with limbs akimbo, pressed in all directions with a little shiver in his toes. Maybe a yawn and a curl of the tongue. When he does this, I call him strange and scratch his ribs, but honestly, I can relate.

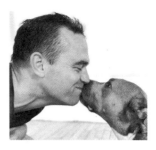

This is the dog in question, by the way. His name is JJ and he's just the worst.

When we sleep, our connective tissue gets dehydrated and sticky; the body's lubrication becomes less viscous, and it's a little harder for layers of tissue to slide over one another. So we get a little stiff. Likewise, in the stillness of sleep, little spiderwebs of collagen—which are always growing inside of us—have an opportunity to bind various tissues together.[48] When we wake up and stretch out, we are opening the internal network of connective tissue back up, loosening these connections, warming and moving the lubrication around, and ridding ourselves of the slight immobility that sleep imposes. This is why a good stretch-and-yawn[49] after a long night is pretty much instinctive for many mammals. It's part of preparing the body for the activity of waking life.

Look at Sun Salutations and you might notice a little bit of this idea. How does it go? Stretch u-u-up, stretch do-o-own, stretch a le-e-eg … You get the picture. The morning routine of greeting the rising sun is, at least in some small part, like the morning stretches of animals both domesticated and wild: wake up, stretch out, say good morning to the sun, get ready. You're here.

In Foundations, we prepare similarly. After what may have been a long period of relative immobility—like a day at an office job—we begin with big, opening shapes. This is the central basis of the first trio of postures: side bends, forward folds, and back bends. When we practice these poses, it can be helpful to think about morning stretches. We're aiming to open up the internal system of connective tissue in preparation for class.

---

[48] Gil Hedley, *Fascia and Stretching: The Fuzz Speech,* video, February 7, 2009, https://youtu.be/_FtSP-tkSug.

[49] A nice dose of extra oxygen to the system wakes you up.

Side Bends

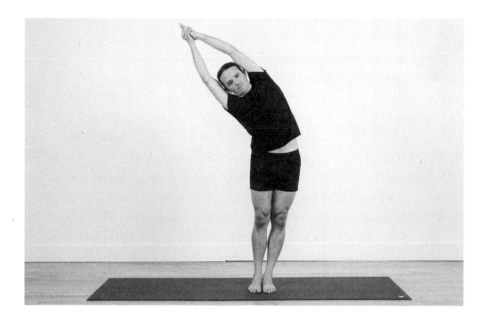

SETUP

With your feet together, take your arms over-head and set a good grip with both hands. (We like Kali Mudra—with your fingers interlaced and the index fingers extended—but there are a bunch more positions available in the options section.)

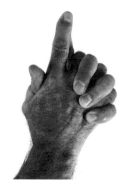

Before you start working too hard, bend your knees slightly. This will release the tension in your legs a bit and give you some space to manipulate the position of your pelvis. Now, tuck your tailbone downward and straighten out your legs again.

Reach your arms high. Be mindful of the position of your rib cage and spine here. You may notice that the ribs want to flare out, causing your mid-back to get compressed. Adjust yourself as necessary; remember Healthy Neutral in the torso is primary here.

JOSEPHINE: ARMS OVERHEAD AND RIB CAGE POSITION (EXERCISE)

Recall that the Josephine tells us to look at things from dual perspectives—holistic and component—so we can understand how things are connected. Let's take a moment here to investigate the integration of the arms and the rib cage.

Stand with your back against a wall, heels touching it. If you don't have a wall, find a tree or a lifeguard stand or the side of a rusted-out VW minibus or something. (If you don't have those things because you're in some sort of formless void, please stop reading. The concepts in this book do not hold up well in formless voids.) Set your mid-back so it's relatively flat against the wall. Now slowly swing your arms up in an arc in front of you, paying close attention to the contact of your back against the wall. You may reach a point at which you have to choose: either lift your arms all the way up or keep your back flat on the wall. It might be unavailable for you to do both at the same time.[50]

Alternatively, put your arms down by your sides and turn your palms forward. With the backs of your hands against the wall, slowly sweep your arms upward in a wide arc. Just like before, you might notice your lower ribs start to poke forward, and you start to back-bend off the wall as your arms reach overhead. You might notice you can go farther than when you brought your arms up in the front plane, or that you can't go as far. That's because you've changed the tension patterns in your shoulders by rotating your arms and lifting them in a different direction.

The position of your arms and the position of your rib cage are deeply interconnected. The orientation and movement of one manipulates the other. It's a pretty basic idea, but it's important to keep in mind as we are

---

[50] By the way, if you can hold your back flat against the wall and get your arms vertical overhead, you have been blessed by the Great Marsupial in the sky, goddess of Humeri. But be cautious, dear traveler; her scorned lover is the patron saint of Downward Facing Dog, a renowned trickster who preys on the hubris of wayward souls.

building yoga poses. "Arms overhead" is a very common position in yoga. We should have a sense of how it affects the practice.

For many human beings, putting their arms over their head vertically is not anatomically possible without imposing a back bend away from Healthy Neutral. The angle between the arm and the torso can only go so far, due to tension patterns (and potentially bone structure) in and around the shoulders. When these people take arms overhead, they may unintentionally *force* themselves into a compressed back bend in the mid-spine. Remember, Healthy Neutral is primary, so what we're doing with the limbs is secondary. So if your arm position is forcing you to back-bend unnecessarily, we should probably change the position of your arms. Which is cool; we got options.

You might benefit from following the "arms overhead" command without the necessity of "arms vertical." Instead, try moving the arms forward a bit, off the vertical line, to restore Healthy Neutral around the spine.

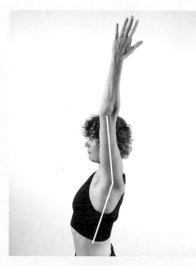 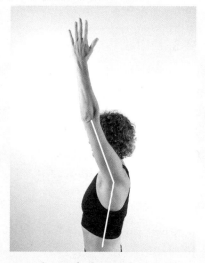

Here, Summer's reaching her arms straight up and tension in her shoulders is driving the top of the rib cage back, which imposes a back bend.

Arms forward of vertical. Notice that the angle between the arms and shoulders hasn't really changed; we are simply choosing to prioritize Healthy Neutral.

I am aware that from a certain perspective this kind of talk might seem trite or overly simplistic. And in a way it is. What I'm saying here could be boiled down to "Your arms are connected to your torso at the shoulders." But it's not just that they are connected, it's about *how* they are connected in your own human body and what that type of connection means. Within a holistic system, how do the components influence one another?

ENTRANCE

Inhale: Stretch up tall.
Exhale: Reach your upper body over to the right and shift your hips left. Your legs should lean sideways off the midline just a bit.

Don't overwork it. Remember, we're just stretching things out to get ready for practice.

ASSESSMENT

Keep the weight over your heels and your toes ungripped from the floor. Many students shift their hips forward and collapse the mid-back in the side bend, releasing the core support necessary to remain in Healthy Neutral. Work to keep the hips back over the heels with the legs straight. It takes real focus and engagement to stabilize the position, but when we do, we can start to explore the integration of leg, hip, and core strength.

BREATHING

Normal breathing is just fine, or you can experiment with moving the breath in different areas of the body. A couple options for this:

1. Breathe into the left side of the ribs—the stretching side—and explore the action of the intercostal muscles as well as their

integration into the obliques. These muscles groups have to coordinate to move breath while supporting the body. It's hard work.

2. Breathe into the right side of the body, where the ribs are compressing into the abdomen. Explore the idea of creating space within compression, intentionally resisting the primary direction of the posture.

OPTIONS

Arm Position: If the arm position or hand grip are not working for you, here are a few alternative positions:

1. Right hand takes left elbow, left arm straight.

2. Hands hold opposite elbows.

3. Left arm straight (as normal), right hand gently grips left side ribs.

   a. In this position, your right hand can provide manual feedback and assistance. Send breath to the point of contact and use your fingertips to spread the tissue on the side of the ribs.

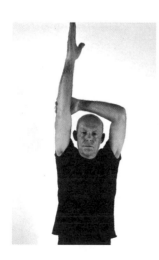 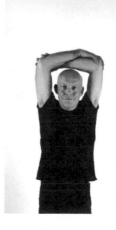 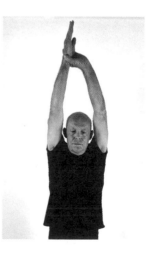

GOALS

1. open the side bodies, left and right.
2. engage and warm up the legs.
3. establish Healthy Neutral inside a simple shape.

DEPTH

In order to keep the side bend from collapsing, we need to integrate the muscle and connective tissue down the whole left side of the body.[51] When well integrated, this line helps hold the side bend in a stable, smooth curve. If one muscle group in the integrated line is weak or inactive, we might see the line "break" into a sharp angle.

For example, when the obliques aren't strong enough to support the torso in the side bend (or they're simply not engaged), we're likely to find the right (lower) side of the rib cage "dropped" into the abdomen and the left side jutting upward.

When this happens, it can be tempting to see the break in the line as a deeper opening, a further development of the posture. And you can choose to see it this way if you like. However, if we are interested in opening and strengthening this line of tissue in a well-integrated fashion, we should adjust the position to correct this collapse in the side body.

Try this: only bend to the side about 50 or 60 percent of what your flexibility allows. Don't fall over; don't pull or drop down. Instead, focus on lifting your heart high away from the ground inside the shape of the side bend. Measure success based on how *long* you can make your spine, not how deeply you can bend it. You will likely discover you can get the same amount of stretch in this position, all while the side body remains stable and engaged.

---

[51] Namely the obliques, serratus anterior, and intercostals, combined with the TFL and gluteus medius, plus their respective connective tissues.

It's not uncommon that our ideas about depth overwhelm our better judgment. When we chase extreme postures we can lose sight of the primary aim of practice, at least as far as this book is concerned, which is the long-term well-being and maintenance of your spectacular, athletic human body.

Keep this theme in mind, we will return to it like Alan Silvestri in *The Avengers*.[52]

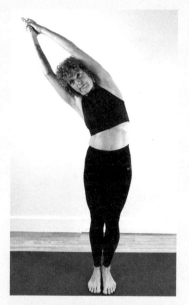 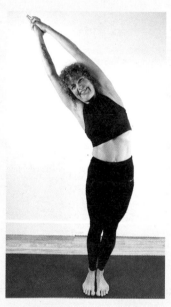

Notice how the right side of Summer's torso is collapsing down and in, and her legs are not leaning to the side.

Here, the side bend is better integrated and her legs are leaning out to the side. Summer is actually leaning over less in this version, but is getting a more complete side body opening.

---

[52] Anybody? Movie score jokes? No? That's fine, I can play with my superhero toys by myself. NBD.

Back Bend

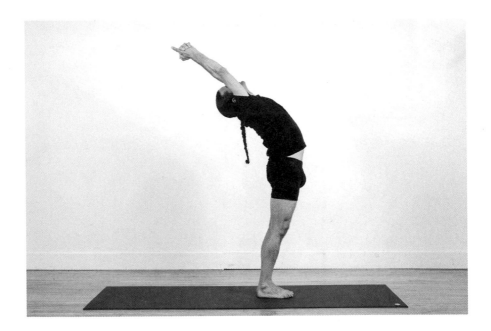

SETUP

Out of the side bends, take a second to do the bend-your-knees, tuck-your-tail, straighten-your-legs-again move to reset the pelvis. I also like to wiggle my head a couple of times to clear extra neck tension.

ENTRANCE

Inhale: Stretch tall.
Exhale: Head drops back gently.
Inhale: Lift your heart.
Exhale: Stay lifted and reach your arms back.

Don't "drop" your body into the back bend. That's too easy. Go back to about 50 to 75 percent of your capacity and—just as in the side bends—think about lifting your heart as high as you can. Make your spine as long as possible. Be sure to breathe. That part is important.[53]

ASSESSMENT

If you're only 50 to 75 percent in this thing, you may find that you're shivering like a meerkat in Siberia right now. That's OK. As long as it's not causing you any pain, keep it up. If we hold the pose back from our end range of motion, we force the muscles to support the posture more. And it turns out that sometimes muscles shake when they're turned on.

The other basics all apply:

+ weight toward the heels

+ unlock your neck

+ soften around the jaw and the tongue

BREATHING

Breathing in a back bend often presents a challenge, particularly when the position is well supported and the abdominal muscles are turned on. All aspects of the torso, front, back, and sides are engaged in stabilizing the body in this rather unusual position. Full breathing in a back bend doesn't just require core strength but the *coordinated movement* of core strength, all while under pressure in an unusual position. When we're beginning, this can be a lot for the body to handle. It's not uncommon for the breathing to get "stuck" in the neck and shoulders during a back bend, especially for beginners, which can increase the emotional stress of the pose and decrease oxygen supply.

---

[53] In a decade teaching, I've had three people faint during my class. One was very hungover (still drunk?), and another had not eaten in nearly twenty-four hours. The third was a very muscular man who held his breath while back-bending. He then briefly attempted to fight me when he came back to consciousness in my arms. True story. Good times. All three totally OK afterward.

RULE OF THREE: LOCALIZED BACK BENDS

When entering into a standing back bend, students sometimes allow them-selves to simply fall backward and release the pose to gravity. This often results in what we call a "localized" back bend, where much of the load of the posture is imposed on a particular portion of the posterior spine. In this position, the back bend is supported largely by compression of the soft tissue and the spinous processes[54] rather than strength. This isn't always bad, but for our purposes—training the body toward Healthy Neutral—we avoid localized back bends. Instead we try to "generalize" our back bends throughout the spine, creating integrated support throughout the torso. We want the whole system to participate.

Doing this in a standing back bend requires a fair degree of abdominal strength. You must prevent yourself from falling backward by *activating forward*. Gravity is doing the bend backward action; you're applying resis-tance. I like to tell people to think about doing a sit-up inside of the back bend to activate the abdominal wall. When you do this, you hold the weight of the torso with muscular strength instead of resting on the compressed bone and tissue of and around the spine.

This work is an example of the Rule of Three in practice: one thing (spinal extension into gravity) combines with its opposite (muscular action toward spinal flexion) and we find the real value of the posture (core stabil-ity in spinal extension) from engaging their resistance.

---

[54] The bumpy protrusions on the back of your spine.

Here's the suggestion: Only go as far as you can without struggling to take a breath. This emphasis on continued breathing might sound a little basic when you say it out loud, but if you pay close attention when you practice, you may discover gripping and gritting and clenching and fighting and turning blue are not that uncommon in your yoga poses. One major reason this occurs is depth chasing: sometimes we push the posture beyond our capacity to breathe evenly. That's not great. Let the breath define the depth, not the other way around. In fact, let's make this a rule for all your poses. We'll even write it down in old-timey script. Ready?

Rule 47012: Breath Defines Depth

Wow—that looks nice. So official. You have my personal permission to get that tattooed wherever you want, by the way. (Well, except that one place.)

OPTIONS

Arm Position: There are some modifications that can make the back bend a little more available in the shoulders and neck. We can also modify the position to find even more core activation, if you're into that kind of thing.

1. If you're still working on the core strength to support your back bend, or it feels like it's "crunching" in your lower back, put your hands on your butt and focus on lifting your heart when you enter the pose.

2. If you want to explore greater activation in the front body and core, interlace your hands behind your head and take your elbows wide as you lean back. Go slow on this one, friend. It's an experience.

GOALS

+ open and activate the front body simultaneously
+ establish stability throughout the legs and hips
+ lengthen the spine in extension
+ begin to open the shoulders

Forward Fold

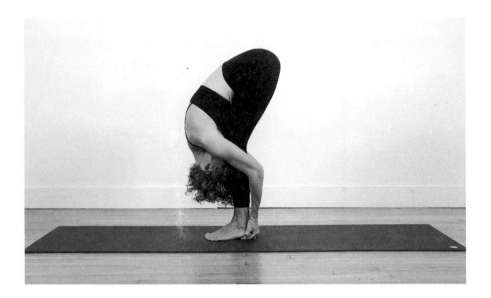

SETUP

Stand up out of the back bend, then buckle your knees and take your hands down toward the floor. (No need to be all fancy about this transition; get there comfortably.) Relax your neck a bit; maybe give your head a gentle shake. Take a load off. Touch your fingertips to the ground and move your shoulders around to loosen them up.

We want to allow your posterior chain to ungrip a bit before we try to lengthen it. For many of us the posterior chain holds excess tension, whether it's in the lower back or the neck or the hamstrings or the feet or … you get the idea. Hopefully we've created some stability through core activation in the back bend, which will help the posterior chain ungrip, but we're not going to force anything. (That's also a rule. Don't force anything. It's, uh … it's rule 485. Sorry, I mean, *Don't force anything.*)

Once you've loosened up a bit, bend your knees more and wrap your hand behind your ankles. You've got the option to slide your hands beneath your feet so your heels fit snugly into the hollows of your palms. Either way is fine. In time, you might work your hands toward each other so their fleshy sides[55] smush against one another.

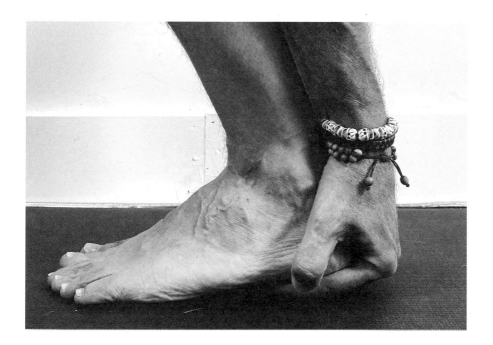

ENTRANCE

Keep the bend in your knees to start, then:

Inhale: Lift your chin, peeling yourself slightly away from your legs.

---

[55] That's your abductor digiti minimi there. Moves your pinkie. Powerful sucker.

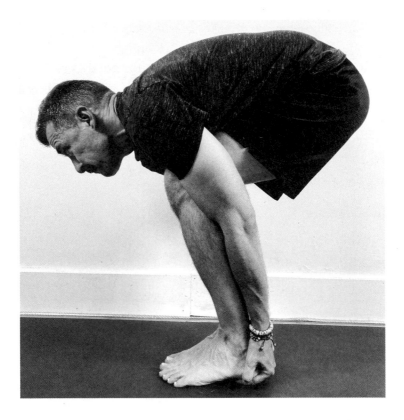

Exhale: Slow and steady, fold your body back onto your legs and begin to pull on your heels, straighten your legs a bit, and gently tuck the chin. Aim your hairline toward your shins.

ASSESSMENT

As we enter into the full fold, it's important to keep in mind this isn't simply a hamstring stretch. Odds are you'll *feel* the hamstrings first; the hamstrings are long and linear and loud, but that shouldn't cloud our approach. If you exclusively target your hamstrings, you might not gain the full benefits of the pose (and you might injure or overstretch the hamstrings). This is a pose for the entire posterior chain, toes to eyebrows.

THE POSTERIOR CHAIN

The posterior chain is, basically, the interwoven line of muscles that runs over the back side of your body.[56] Most importantly this chain includes your calves, hamstrings, glutes, lats, traps, rear deltoids, and erector spinae, and their associated connective tissue. It is occasionally referred to as the "powerhouse of the body" because it is central to your ability to generate force, particularly when you're walking or running around.

When you walk or run, you perform two basic actions: swing and stance. Your swing phase happens whenever your foot is not planted on the ground, or generally when you bring your leg forward. Your stance phase is when your foot is planted, or generally when you push your

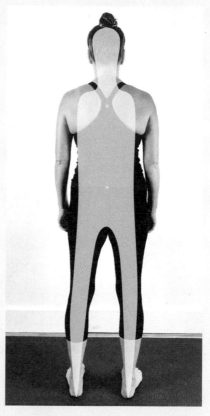

The general lines of the posterior chain, from under the feet, past the heels, up the legs, to the top of the head (and over the skull to the eyebrows).

---

[56] FYI there is some disagreement about what the *posterior chain* means. I prefer a fairly comprehensive definition, which includes (but is also more than) the superficial back line defined by Thomas Myers in *Anatomy Trains*. That's what I'll refer to here. Some others describe a more limited chain that runs from hamstrings to shoulders.

leg (and the ground) backward. While there's no dividing the body neatly—remember the Josephine—we can generally say that your swing phase is a primarily front body action: force from the anterior chain[57] lifts your leg and moves it forward. And generally, your stance phase is a posterior chain action: your glutes, hamstrings, calves, and back muscles coordinate to create "drive" so your body can move forward.

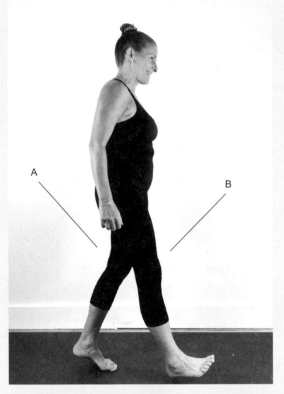

A

B

Stance phase (A) and swing phase (B) during a nice walk across a yoga mat.

---

[57] In this case we are thinking most about abs, quads, and hip flexors. For the most part. It's way more complicated than this—people make whole careers out of studying walking and gait. We're just going for the super basic concepts here.

While both of these actions require energy, the stance phase is primarily responsible for the actual propulsion of your body through space. You get your body—a heavy object, no matter who you are—to move forward by pushing the ground backward. In a healthy gait, this push is primarily generated by the posterior chain, rooted in hip extension.

Hip extension is arguably the most important physical action when it comes to a human body generating power. Standing up from a seat or squat, walking, running, climbing, jumping—they all are rooted largely in hip extension. (Sometimes in combination with extension of the spine in a sort of "spring" motion, like when a long-jumper leaps forward through the air.) This isn't to say other important stuff isn't happening, but if you had to choose the central action for generating power in the world, hip extension would be a decent choice.

Hip flexion, which brings your leg forward by closing the angle of the hip joint, is also vital to healthy movement. However, it's not the main way humans generate drive when they walk or run, so it doesn't need to be quite as powerful.

What this means is that a well-functioning human body, at least in terms of evolutionary design, generates more power from its posterior than anterior side. (There's a reason you don't have a butt on the front side of your body. Which is a terrible image; I'm so sorry, but it's actually pretty telling when you think about it. So … don't think about it too long. Just think about it long enough to get the point and then immediately stop thinking about it forever.) When in Healthy Neutral, your body meets this need for power through the integration and coordination of the entire posterior chain.

Imagine a single elastic cord running from your eyebrows, over the back of your skull, down your spine, all the way under your feet to the bottoms of your toes. If you were to tighten that cord, its entire length would reflect this increase in tension. Tugging at the top of the cord will pull on the bottom of the cord, and vice versa. Your posterior chain has a sort of similar quality:[58] pulling on one part has reverberative effects throughout the chain.

One way to explore this quality during a forward fold is to assess your neck tension and head position. When you enter the fold, do you find that the back of your neck is tight? Are you staring at the floor? (Also: is the stare aggressive? Are you establishing dominance over your yoga mat? Is it working?) Notice that the shape of the pose here tightens the posterior chain by drawing it to its full length, so you may begin to experience a small tug at the back of your skull. If you gently tuck your chin and aim your hairline to the shins, you lengthen and tighten this chain further. As a result, tucking your chin may make you feel a stretch elsewhere in the posterior chain. (Personally, I feel it in my mid-back, but it can show up all over, depending on your individual patterns. Sometimes it pops up all the way down by the hips; sometimes it never gets below the level of the neck.) What we're trying to illustrate here is the connection between the position of your skull and the tension of a chain of tissue that runs down your whole back body.

This is a sort of "tell." It's not an automatic sign of an absolute condition, but it shows that something might be happening. An unconscious gripping in the back of the neck is often—though not always—a reflection of tension throughout the posterior chain. This tension could be structural (the tissue is short and tight) emotional (stress response) or both.

This isn't exclusive to the neck. It shows up all over the chain. Toes gripping the mat? That's a shortening of the chain in your feet. Weight shifting back from the toes? Slight plantarflexion in the ankle, friend; that's probably your calves shortening. The point is, if we think of the posterior chain as a holistic unit, we can investigate how adjustments in one place manipulate other points in the system.

---

[58] I say "sort of" because it's not that simple or uniform. You can, of course, move portions of the chain with relative independence. It is both a collection of components and a holistic, interconnected line.

Standing, walking, and running patterns benefit from a posterior chain that is both mobile and strong. If the posterior chain is weak (along with the abdominal wall) you may start to "rest" the weight of the torso on the bones of the spine, warping it away from Healthy Neutral. This can lead us into patterns of kyphosis or lordosis or a mixture of both. If the posterior chain is stiff, it limits our access to a wide range of movements. (For example, if you have ever tweaked your back, you know how limited day-to-day life is when the posterior chain can't move without pain.) Maladaptive body patterns almost always involve some sort of combination of excess tension and a lack of strength in the posterior chain.

The standing forward fold—along with Intense West Stretch, which is essentially the same pose flipped 90 degrees—is the most direct and comprehensive opening of the posterior chain that you can get. There isn't really a position you can get into that will lengthen this chain more completely. This is, of course, not the only thing going on in the pose, but it's primary and worth digging into.

With this sort of investigation, we're working our way toward a more holistic concept of the body as an integrated system.

According to the Rule of Three, we're going to apply an opposite to the forward fold. We did this in the back bend as well, turning on the abdominal muscles—some of the more prominent "forward bend" muscles—while going backward. Now, going forward, we will apply the back benders.

It goes like this: without shortening your neck again, gently begin to draw your shoulder blades toward your hips. (So, since you're inverted, toward the ceiling or the sky.) Imagine, perhaps, gently doing a back bend like Cobra pose inside the forward fold. Imagine the back body *shortening,* even as it draws longer. We're effectively activating the stretch of your posterior chain, engaging the same muscles we are lengthening.

Activating the muscles you are lengthening, called isometric stretching, is one of the best ways to safely increase flexibility and can help us restore balance to anterior or posterior tension patterns in the body.

BREATHING

Take smooth, full, gentle breaths. Allow the inhales to expand into the back body. You might explore a slight chin tuck as you exhale.

BACK BREATHING

Our default thinking about breath is often front-body oriented. Even our standard language of "chest breathing" and "belly breathing" belies our bias toward the front side. And while these areas tend to move the *most* when we breathe, they are certainly not the *only* places where the breath moves. The back of your rib cage and your lower back are deeply involved in the process of taking a breath, for starters. Keep in mind, your respiratory diaphragm connects to your lower back more substantially than it does the front side of your body.

Teaching your back to breathe fully is a powerful practice and can help reshape the way your body holds tension. It can help pattern core stability and mobility of tissue in the back. In my experience, intentional breathing is arguably the safest, most effective way to unlock excessive tension in the posterior chain.

In a forward fold we are effectively eliminating belly breathing, as the abdomen is pressed firmly against the thighs, and greatly limiting the capacity for breath in the front of the chest. In order to take a full breath here, we *need* to access the back body. For some of us this will be easier said than done. It's not uncommon to experience the fold as somewhat stressful, as the breath might be forced to the top of the chest, and perhaps the neck begins to grip. The first step toward unlocking the breath in the back is just to notice what's going on there. Notice if you are holding any stress tension that you may not need.

Once you have let go of unneeded tension, imagine the back-body pulsing like great wings beating in slow motion. Picture them swelling out from the centerline of the spine, then gathering back again. Inhale and exhale. Let breath determine depth, here. If you are struggling with the breath or just fighting the posture in general, back away from it a bit. Keep your mind on this idea; opening and closing the back muscles like wings. Over time this idea can translate into action, and so a concept becomes practice, and practice becomes pattern, and pattern becomes the next action.

OPTIONS

1. If wrapping your hands behind your legs doesn't work for you, it's fine to just touch the floor or gently hold your ankles.

2. Keeping feet together doesn't work for some people. This can be because of body type, pelvic structure, general tension patterns, or foul mood. It's completely acceptable to take your feet out to the width of your hips, or wider if you choose. This is a very "big" shape; there is tension throughout a major physical chain. Make the adjustments that feel right for you.

GOALS

♦ open the posterior chain
♦ establish breathing in the back body

Power Sequence

The Power Sequence is a combination of chair variations and lunging poses. We use it as part of the warm-up; it gets the legs, hips, glutes, and core muscles engaged and activated in preparation for the full class.

We do three chair variations here: a traditional chair with the arms up and slight spinal extension, a chair on the toes with the spine upright, and Power Pose, with the spine rounded in flexion. Then we move to a high lunge and add a revolve at the end. Altogether we perform four of the six motions of the spine (no side bends) on top of leg-strengthening poses.

So it's a whole thing.

Chair Pose

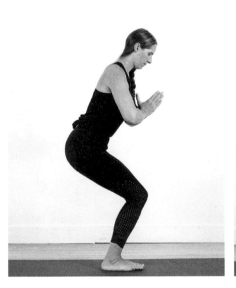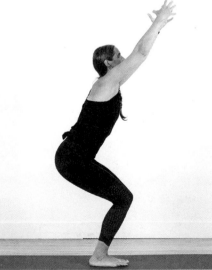

SETUP

Start with hands in prayer with your feet together, with just a little space between your heels. Bend your knees slightly so you can squeeze your thighs against one another, then shift your weight to your heels. Keep the weight there as we continue to build the pose. This part is hard and requires focus, but that's cool. We don't practice yoga to check out, right?

ENTRANCE

Inhale: Lift your chest.
Exhale: Sit your hips down and back, driving the weight of the body back through the heels.

Try not to let your knees move too far past your toes. We want to load the posture back into the hips instead of forward into the knees.

Once you're down, drop your chin a bit and look to the floor to unlock your neck. Then move your head back to align it with your shoulders, and breathe deeply, head to hips. If we have your neck lined up, your hips back behind your heels, and your core well supported, this thing is probably already a challenge.

ASSESSMENT

- legs together strongly
- spine at Healthy Neutral
- heels heavy, toes soft
- belly strong

There are a few cheats that show up a lot in this Chair Pose. A big one, which we will see regularly, is hyperextension of the thoracolumbar spine: the mid-back sinks into a localized back bend. This happens usually when we don't have effective core support from the abdominal wall; it's easier for your body to hang its weight on the back of the spine than it is to support that weight with abdominal strength. So it hangs.

Make sure you're maintaining strong abdominal support as you sit into the chair. If you get to a certain depth and you feel like you *must* sink into the lower back to go any farther, maybe just stop there. Do what's available.

Also, notice your neck. Keep checking in there to make sure it is not locked.[59] Healthy Neutral is a whole-spine action. If the neck is locked in hyperextension, we will probably lose integration through the whole torso. Check for tension: neck, jaw, teeth, tongue, roof of the mouth, base of the skull.

CHEATS

Remember the "efficiency machine" idea? Unless it's made to do otherwise, your body is going to use its existing habits and strength patterns to support yoga poses, so we have to be aware of where and how that happens. In many cases, reverting to your habits means you avoid the good work of a yoga pose. This is what we call a "cheat."

A common cheat is to simply sink the weight of the body onto a joint, allowing the muscles around the joint to relax a bit. One example of this is knee locking. When we take the knee all the way to extension the joint "locks" and the muscles around it can disengage. This is an evolved trait; your body doesn't want to spend unnecessary energy just standing around, so we developed this standing position where we dropped into the joint. And this is just fine for short periods of time, especially when the muscles around the joint are strong.

In order to rest into a joint, it must be at its end range of motion, like when your knees are locked or you're "hanging" on your shoulders in Downward-Facing Dog. At this end range, the connective tissue is the primary source of stability, so your muscles don't have to kick on as much. When you go to your

---

[59] The neck does not actually "lock" like a knee; it grips tightly in hyperextension and immobilizes the skull. So they're not physiologically the same action, but the result is similar.

end range of motion in yoga poses, taking your joints all the way to their limits, you are potentially making the pose *easier* in terms of muscular engagement.

It's helpful to look for places where the posture "sinks" into a joint and the muscles around it are disengaged. Odds are that, to some degree, the body is resting on the connective tissue in that place. This isn't always a bad thing; sometimes we want to put weight on the connective tissue to create tension. Sometimes that's just the way people choose to practice. But we can't really make an intelligent determination if something is a "cheat" until we know what we are looking for. In Foundations we almost always try to avoid sitting too heavily into any particular joint. Instead, we focus on creating healthy support structures around the bones through balanced tension.

When you find a cheat and want to fix it, try to engage a healthy boundary of strength around the joint. (Basically, turn the muscles on.) This usually requires you back away from the joint's end range of motion, for example, bending a locked knee a bit. Once you've come back from the brink—from depth—you may find you can explore muscle activation and joint support with a little more control and detail.

If you've got a lot of tension in your lower back, but weak glutes, you might (unconsciously) adjust your Chair Pose so your lower back is the main support structure for the pose. And while you could probably hold your Chair Pose longer this way, in the long term you'd miss out on one of its major benefits: strong glutes. Which is sad.

One way to look for cheats is to work intently on the details of your poses, assessing them constantly for habitual patterns and making adjustments accordingly. Another way is to just feel your body. If you're doing a yoga pose with the intention of making your glutes stronger, but you don't feel your glutes turning on? That's a sign that the load of the pose is probably being carried elsewhere.

BREATHING

Experiment with moving the breath through the back of the torso, all the way to the hips. If this sounds weird, just imagine the breath as a wave on the ocean. The muscles of your back are the surface of the water. You might not feel it at first; that's cool. Just hold that image and don't push too hard. Have patience, cricket; we're learning.

In time, focus on deepening the exhales.

OPTIONS

If you have all of the assessment stuff in order and the pose isn't falling apart, you might explore adding to the pose.

* Lift your arms up overhead like you're presenting a very important beach ball to a demanding toddler in the clouds. Then pause. Notice if the back of your neck has started to lock up or if your ribs are pressing forward. If so, that's a sign your body may be trying to cheat by dropping into a localized backbend. Keep your neck long, your spine neutral, your weight in the heels, and your breathing steady.

* If you can keep the neck from gripping, start to look up. This is a great moment for personal assessment. From the outside, teachers can't always tell if your neck is locked when you're looking up. So, you've got to feel it. Does it *feel* like you've started locking the back of your neck? Your call. If you feel a lot of tension behind the skull, then try taking your chin back down to line up your skull again.

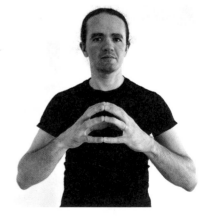

Isaiah holding the sphere.

* Hold the sphere: you might try touching all the fingertips

of both hands together, like you're holding a big grapefruit or a small armadillo out in front of you. This can help open your shoulders a bit, which can come in handy when we're trying to adjust your ribs and core and pelvis and, oh, no, now we're talking about the whole body again.

 ◆ If standing with your feet together doesn't work for you, spread your feet to about hip width and put a block between your knees.[60]

GOALS

 ◆ strengthen glutes, thighs, and ankles

 ◆ engage and strengthen adductors

 ◆ decompress spine, particularly through "back breathing"

 ◆ strengthen core muscles in neutral alignment

 ◆ warm up the body and raise the heart rate

---

[60] What we're going for here is active engagement of your adductors—the inner thigh muscles—which are vital for pelvic stability and a healthy gait, and also can become weak with a sedentary lifestyle. (When humans sit down, they often do so with their knees turned out. This is a disengaged position for the adductors.) Squeezing the knees or thighs together or block-hugging creates resistance, which makes the adductors reengage.

Chair on Toes

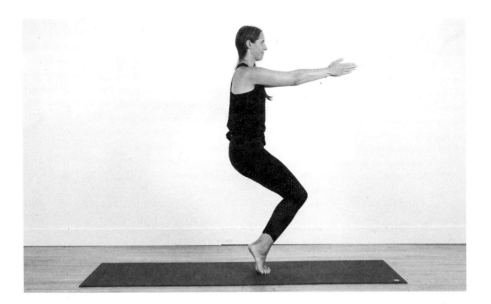

SETUP

Stand up from Chair Pose until your legs are almost straight. Keep a little bend so your knees and thighs can stay together. Point your arms straight forward of your heart, palms together. Push the balls of the feet down through the mat and slowly lift your heels high off the floor.

ENTRANCE

Sit down toward that imaginary chair again, high on the balls of the feet. Only sit down as low as you can with your torso upright.

ASSESSMENT

Setup for Chair on Toes.

Balls of the feet anchored: many people have challenges with ankle stability, so the load collapses into the outer ankles. Notice if the line of your shin is consistent with the line of your feet. If they're not in a relatively straight line, you may be collapsing a bit into the outer ankles. To fix this, imagine there's a big, pudgy marmot between your ankles and give it a generous hug. (If it helps, this marmot's name is Lawrence and he's a Pisces.)

Torso upright: it's a lot easier to do this pose if you lean forward, as it relieves the strength work in your hips and thighs especially. So, you know, don't do that. The moment your torso wants to pitch forward, slow everything down. This can occasionally be an ego check, because you may not get as low as you think you "should." Sour grapes, friend. Remember, we want to choose building the new pattern over reinforcing the old one.

Check for tension: send your attention to your neck, jaw, teeth, tongue, roof of your mouth, and base of your skull.

Shoulders neutral: not up in your ears, for one. But also, there's no need to force them down. Maybe give them a little shimmy and let them settle on their own.

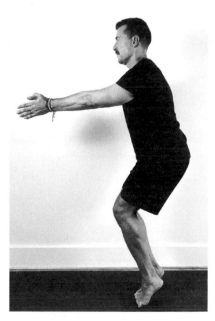 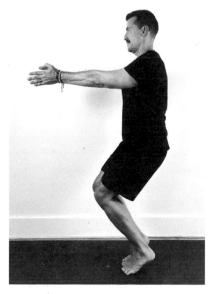

Don't do this.   *Do this.*

Neutral position of the skull: notice if your head is pushed forward of neutral, or the back of the neck is squeezed tight. Go easy here. Let your head float back and see if you can get it lined up nicely over the rib cage.

Put on the seatbelt.

THE SEATBELT

The Seatbelt is a metaphor, not a literal anatomical structure (and even if it were, it wouldn't have this name, because most major body structures were given their names before seatbelts were invented,[61] and anyways there's no Latin word for seatbelt because the ancient Romans were exceptionally cautious drivers.)

When we lose core stability, we may sometimes end up with a standing body pattern where the femurs are externally rotated and the lower abdomen falls down and forward. To correct this—and the patterns associated with it—we imagine a line going from one ASIS[62] to the other, about two inches below the level of the navel. Right about where a seatbelt would go.

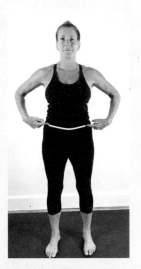

The Seatbelt.

Now imagine tightening that seatbelt, point to point, across your waist. You may notice the navel gently tones back and up, the tailbone scoops down, and the femoral heads draw forward a bit. Hopefully, we are relieving tension in the lower back and sacrum here, drawing the bottom of the spine into a more stable position.

---

[61] Note to self: Research seatbelts on horse-drawn buggies. Were those a thing?

[62] Anterior superior iliac spine, what many of us call the "hip bones" where your pelvis protrudes toward the front of either hip. You may be able to feel these bones easily on your own body; you may not. Regardless, it is often helpful to know where they are located on your own personal skeleton.

BREATHING

Full-torso breathing. Squeeze your thighs together, soften your jaw, and send an inhale from the sinuses to the lower back. As you exhale, gently tighten the seatbelt.

OPTIONS

- Hands "hold the sphere."
- Block between the knees, if thighs together doesn't feel good for you.
- Remember, only go down as far as you can staying upright. If this means you only bend your knees a tiny bit, that's fine. Take your time and work toward greater depth with patience and attention to detail.

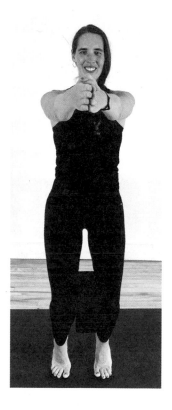

GOALS

- strengthen glutes, thighs, calves, and ankles
- engage and strengthen adductors
- open plantar fascia
- wake up the brain-body connection through balance
- aid in spinal decompression, particularly with "back breathing"
- strengthen core muscles in neutral alignment
- warm up the body and raise the heart rate

Power Pose

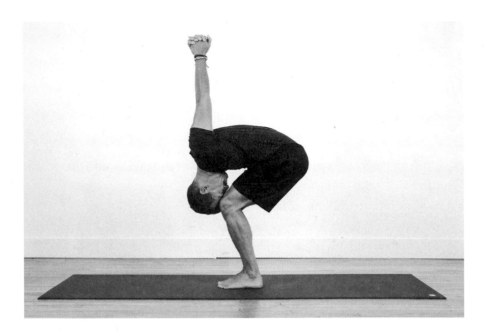

SETUP AND ENTRANCE

This one has what we called a "pulse" entrance, where we coordinate motion and breath to get the pose into shape. In this approach, the setup and entrance are pretty much the same thing. It goes like this. Starting from the previous position, up on your toes:

Inhale: Fully, nice and slow.
Exhale: Gently drop your heels to the mat and fall toward a forward fold. Interlace your hands behind your back for a shoulder stretch. (If you like, you might stay in this position for a few breaths.)

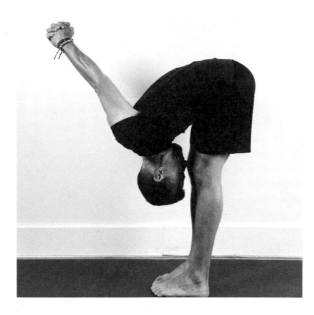

Inhale: Lift your chest to look forward and sit your hips low into an imaginary chair.

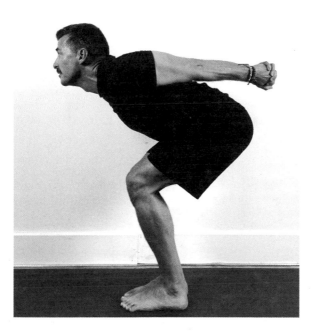

Exhale: Staying low in the chair, round your spine and try to touch your forehead to your knees.

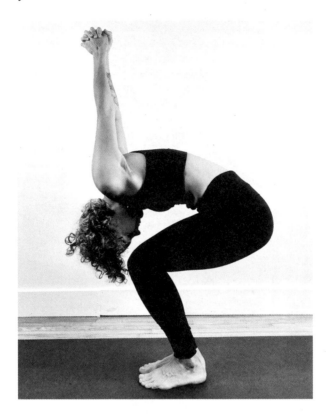

Depending on body type and tension patterns, many people can't actually touch the head to the knees here. That's cool. What we're trying to do is round the spine in a chair position as best we can.

Keep breathing the whole time. Breathing will help you reorganize the tension patterns in your torso, and has the added benefit of keeping you alive.

ASSESSMENT

◆ Weight toward the heels.

◆ Arms lifting up to a manageable shoulder stretch. You can bend your elbows or separate the palms if that feels better. Don't force anything: just work on taking the shoulders back and the hands up as much as feels comfortably available.

◆ Tuck your chin. This one is really annoying, but try it out if you can. What usually happens is your body wants to cheat and use back tension instead of abdominal support to hold this pose. That back tension pulls on your neck, because your neck is functionally an extension of your back. This "pull" makes the back of the neck short, so now maybe you're staring at the ground with your eyebrows up and probably a deep, fiery loathing for whatever this stupid pose is.

◆ Go easy. Just pull your belly in, tuck your chin a bit, and breathe. It'll be more difficult physically, but you might find a whole bunch of *emotional* resistance melts away. We're going to find this with neck tension a lot. If we can let emotional resistance go, the poses get much more manageable.

BREATHING

The deep work in Power Pose is to balance strengthening the abdominal muscles with opening the muscle and fascia of the back. Send your inhales into your back as much as is available, and use your exhales to tone your navel to your spine. This will require focus and engagement. At first it may be only a thought. That's all right; keep working with that thought. With practice, thinking about it will turn into feeling it. When we apply intention over time, things start to shift.

KIDNEY WINGS

One of my favorite anatomical images is that of the Kidney Wings[63] areas of the back, where the rib cage meets the lower back. They're so-named because they're in the general location of the kidneys, on the posterior portion of the body right around the lowest ribs. This area—around the thoracolumbar junction—is the most mobile spot on your spine outside your neck. Because this area is so mobile, it is susceptible to maladaptive patterns, often involving compression or gripping around the kidney wings.

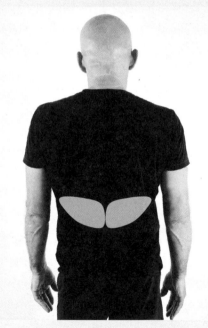

Robert with some really impressive kidney wings.

---

[63] Full disclosure, this isn't my image. I heard it in a class in Colorado, almost as a throwaway line like a jillion other yoga metaphors. But it stuck with me, so now I've decided it's a big deal. Maybe everyone west of the Mississippi says it. Maybe there's a really cool post-postmodern vinyasa studio in Santa Monica called Kidney Phoenix that holds transcendental movement classes and angel-themed séances every solstice, and whose apparel is designed by Banksy, and sometimes Kate Beckinsale goes there. I don't know. I didn't google it. I'm just saying I didn't invent the term.

So try this real quick. Sit or stand upright and inhale as deeply as you can into your kidney wings. Imagine them spreading slowly as you do. Then as you exhale, let them slowly fall.

Focusing on the kidney wings is a way to access to back-body breathing, the expansion of the posterior ribs, and core engagement on the inhale. You may find that focusing on the motion of the kidney wings in particular, and the whole back in general, allows for fuller, more engaged breath in nearly all of your yoga postures.

Keep this idea in mind. It'll pop up all over.

Power Pose is tough. Don't push your body any farther than it can go while maintaining the pulse of the breath. Remember, Breath Defines Depth.

OPTIONS

- Hands don't have to be bound. If your shoulders get resistant or you feel tweaky, you can put your hands on your hips. Use this hand position to encourage your pelvis to tuck under, rounding the spine more.

- You can make it more challenging by reaching your arms straight out in front of you, as close to parallel to the floor as you can. Keep your chin tucked, spine rounded, and hips low. This variation turns into a real situation about 0.7 seconds into the process, so take your time with it.

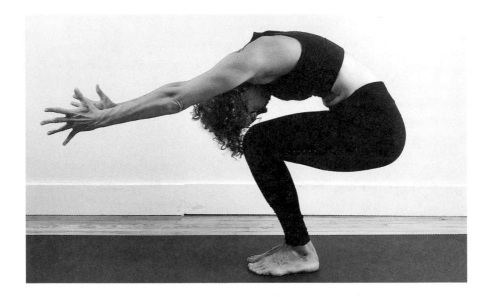

GOALS

- strengthen glutes, thighs, and ankles
- engage and strengthen adductors
- engage and strengthen abdominal wall
- open the tissue of the back
- open the shoulders (with hands bound)
- encourage mindful breathing
- warm up the body and raise the heart rate

Revolved Lunge

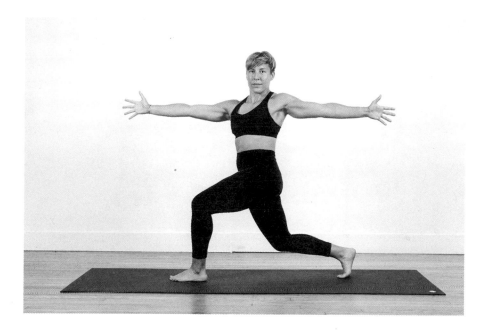

SETUP

From Power Pose, look at the mat. Lift your left foot off the floor, heel toward your butt (BTW FYI "butt" is an actual anatomical term, it's in books, so I'm allowed).

Slowly step your left foot back to a lunge. Slower is harder here. The longer you take to extend your leg back and touch it to the mat, the more challenging you will find the motion. Do what works for you.

Once you have touched down in the lunge, lift your chest up and bend your back knee.

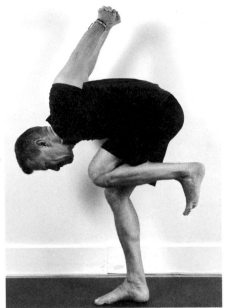

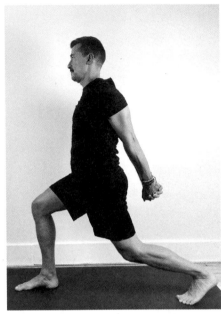

Then lift your arms up to complete the high lunge. You might be tempted here to drive your left leg straight, especially if you're a flexible yoga type, but maintain a healthy bend there. Remember, one of the ways we avoid cheats is to back away from the full range of motion in the joints. When you bend your back knee, you'll find your leg and hip muscles have to engage to keep you stable. That's good; that's what we're after.

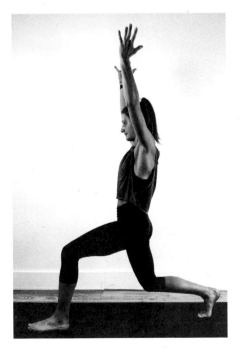

ENTRANCE

Inhale: Get tall through the spine and reach high through the fingertips. Anchor your right heel.

Exhale: Point both arms forward and knit your ribs back.

It's very common to arrive at this pose with the rib cage jutting forward.

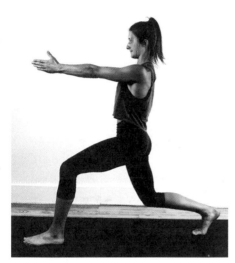 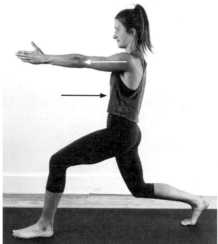

Reach your arms forward and draw the ribs back with this exhale, setting the spine toward neutral.

Inhale: Draw your right hand back to your heart like you're pulling a bow.

Exhale: Turn your chest to the right. Stretch your right arm back and your left arm forward. Keep your hips relatively square to the front of your mat and level to the ground. Look to the right side.

ASSESSMENT

Check for tension: neck, jaw, teeth, tongue, roof of the mouth, base of the skull (are we noticing a pattern here?)[64]

- Align your back foot vertically, with the heel pointing upward and the toes down.

- Keep the weight in your heel on the front foot, and ungrip your toes from the mat.

- Track the line of your right knee. Try not to let it drift inward of the ankle (to the left, if your right foot is forward). Work on setting the tibia—your shin bone—at a clean vertical line.

- Open the line of the heart, first shoulder to shoulder, but then eventually hand to hand and fingertips to fingertips.

- Set your pelvis under your heart with the pelvic bowl relatively level all around, at Healthy Neutral. You might notice the pelvis tries to tilt forward or spin the left side forward. Keep that in mind. It doesn't have to be fixed perfectly, but play with the idea. You'll probably find that rearranging the orientation of the pelvis creates entirely new and different demands on your leg muscles. New patterns, actions, and orientations that are not habitual to us create new forms of strength.

We're creating an exaggerated running stance, in a way, with an open-chain, contralateral rotation (right knee forward, right arm back) and a long stride.

---

[64] I used to tell people to "check your neck" in class, until someone informed me that this is a well-used term in the U.S. South. Apparently, "Check your neck" has close ties to the derogatory use of the term *redneck* and means something like "Please take a moment to notice that you're being a bit of a redneck right now, friend. Perhaps you should practice a bit more social awareness. We don't want to upset the yuppies."

FALL-RUNNING

Every summer a marathon passes through the middle of my town.[65] I love watching it. It's a wonderful opportunity to get outside and cheer for my neighbors and drink coffee and marvel at a sort of discipline and endurance I do not myself have.

Recently, I began to notice something at the marathon: about 45 percent of the runners were fall-running. That is to say, they were doing this thing where they leaned their upper bodies forward, hunched their shoulders, and swung their arms in little circles in front of their torsos like shadowboxers as they jogged down the road. The orientation of their torsos was more downward than upright, their hearts and eyes pointed at the ground about eight feet in front of them. It was as if they were falling toward the ground with every step, only to swing a leg forward just in time to catch themselves and keep moving on.

This running style is essentially a repeated process of falling-catching-falling-catching, over and over. The stance phase of this stride occurs almost entirely on the anterior plane, in front of the body, and the hips never move into full extension. Basically, there's not much backward "kick" to the stride.

If you watch people fall-running, you may notice they rarely have well-defined glutes.[66] When you fall-run there's not much hip extension. You don't move your legs back with much power. And if you're not moving your stance phase *behind you*, you're probably not using the full power of your posterior chain.

This is a pattern, a positive feedback loop that can often involve things like chairs and phones. In terms of a story, it might look like this: I sit on my

---

[65] I wrote this sentence before the summer of 2020 when, for reasons, we did not have said marathon. So not *every* summer but ... you know ... every *semi-normal* summer.

[66] Don't ogle. Don't make it weird.

butt all day long and my butt and hamstrings lose tone. Since they're not very strong, I use the front side muscles (hip flexors and quads, especially) more than my glutes and hamstrings when I run. Since I use my quads and hip flexors, they get more powerful while my glutes and hamstrings continue to lose tone (from more sitting and less activation). Also, since I sit in hip flexion, my body starts to develop a hip flexion pattern, much like how my elbow might pattern in flexion if I wore a sling on my arm for hours a day. This can become deeply ingrained if I don't take the time to counterbalance it. Over time, this front-back, flexion-extension imbalance fundamentally changes my running style and makes me a fall-runner.

Compare fall-running to elite running and you'll see some important differences in body type and form. Elite runners—the people who *win* the marathon[67]—hold their torsos upright in Healthy Neutral, move their legs behind them in their stance phase, and have very powerful posterior chains. (Generally, sprinters are more apparently powerful in their glutes than marathon runners because of muscle type and training style, but the overall idea is the same for both.) Their eyes and hearts are pointed to the horizon, not down in front of them.

Fall-runners (very generally) use existing, anterior chain–dominant patterns when they move, so their torsos lean forward into a hunched position. (If you look closely, you might notice a chair-pattern in fall-runners, they sometimes assume a kind of "hunched at a desk while jogging" shape in their bodies.) We can address this pattern when we practice lunges of all kinds, as long as we're paying attention. Think about those sprinters, upright and strong with powerful core muscles, while you do your lunges. Healthy Neutral in the pelvis and lower back is particularly helpful. If you practice with this in mind, you may find a stronger, more challenging pose that opens and stabilizes healthy walking and running patterns.

---

[67] Not that it's a competition. Which it definitely is.

OPTIONS

To increase the opening across the shoulders and chest, place your back hand behind your head and draw the elbow wide. Then make a strong fist with your front hand and push it away like you're very slowly punching a designer handbag.

GOALS

- strengthen glutes, thighs, and ankles
- support hip stability
- open plantar fascia of the back foot
- lengthen hip flexor of the back leg side
- stabilize open chain rotation: activate and strengthen rotational muscles, particularly the transverse abs
- decompress the spine, particularly with full breath during rotation
- warm up the body and raise the heart rate

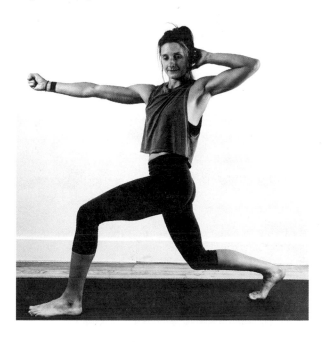

Balancing Sequence

N ow that we've completed the warm-up, we are ready to move on to more challenging postures. The Balancing positions require powerful focus and teach you to engage unusual and underused body patterns, particularly in terms of hip stability.

Eagle

SETUP

From arms overhead, cross your right arm under your left, at the elbows, and then cross the wrists as well.[68] Sit down like Chair Pose and then step your right leg back in a half lunge stance, then bring your weight firmly to your left heel. Push that heel down firmly and feel your left hip engage. You might let this sink in; notice the direct connection between your heel on the floor and your hip.[69]

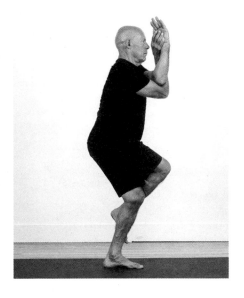

---

[68] I'm desperately trying to avoid overexplaining this. If you're new to Eagle, it can be weirdly hard to understand the arm position, and you should probably ask a teacher to help you out. There may be good videos on YouTube. The written word is a poor substitute here. When you know how to do it, nothing could be easier. So … just cross your arms in Eagle, OK?

[69] In the study of human anatomy, this connection is often referred to as the "leg."

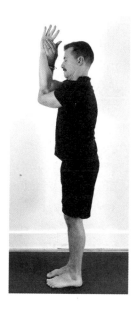
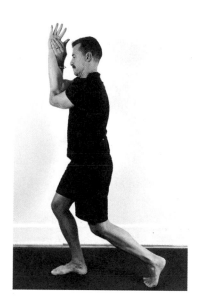

ENTRANCE

Maintaining that connection of the floor, the heel, and the hip, step your right leg up high in front of you, then cross it over your left leg.

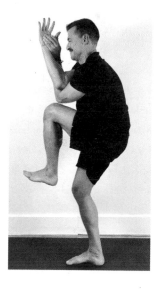
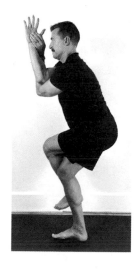

Many of you may have an established practice where you cross the right foot behind the left calf or ankle as well, but we're going to hold off on that here. Instead, simply try to get your right shin parallel to your left and point your toes at the ground. Why, you ask? Isn't Eagle done with that extra little leg cross maneuver? Well, yes. Normally.

Once you're set up, sit your hips down and back.

ASSESSMENT

There's a great deal going on with Eagle. Unusual positions impose unusual demands. As in the forward fold, we are opening the back body and restricting the front. Except this time, we're doing this opening outward from the midline (laterally) and not up and down the postural chain. Think of returning your shoulder blades to the midline of the back, even as they are drawn away from it via the arm position.

BINDS

In the "standard" version of Eagle people wrap their foot behind the opposite ankle. This can be helpful in developing mobility in the hips, but I've found that once students are capable of performing this "bind" it can become a bit of a crutch. While bound up, it's pretty easy to let the posture sit into the joints without really activating the muscles in the thighs and hips. In a certain sense, it can encourage cheating.

Here's something to try. If you're entering the practice and you're unable to wrap your lifted foot behind the other ankle, then work in that direction studiously until you can. But then, once this maneuver becomes available, start to shorten the amount of time you hold it there. In my practice, I wrap my foot into the "bind" and settle into the pose for one long breath. Then I slowly take the foot out of the "bind" while keeping it as close to my ankle as possible.

This is hard, but it helps maintain mobility in the hips before switching into a more challenging, strength-focused shape.

Likewise, you might imagine the outer hips moving in toward the sacrum, against the internal rotation in the thighs imposed by the position.

+ Do your best to send breath into the kidney wings, even as you lift your chest and elbows.

+ Keep the back of the neck long and the jaw soft. Notice if you're starting to lift the shoulder blades up toward your skull, or vice versa, and adjust toward Healthy Neutral with the back of the neck long and the shoulders settled down gently on the back body.

+ Ground through your heel into the floor and try to keep your knee from moving too far beyond the line of your toes. This one is hard, particularly because we don't often have a visual line (unless you're standing sideways at a full-length mirror, in which case you've got it easy), and the "cheat" away from really using your glutes can be deeply ingrained. Do what's available and hold back on the depth. In time you'll develop enough combined strength and mobility to sit farther into the posture without driving the knee forward.[70]

BREATHING

Explore the potential of breathing into your back, as in the forward fold. Especially notice that the angle of the arms has drawn the upper back taut around the back of the rib cage, and restricts the motion of the upper chest. While the breath may drop into the belly fairly easily here, try stabilizing the torso and moving the pulse of breath to the kidney wings.

---

[70] Quick note: A friend of mine is an accomplished trainer who has spent years working on best practices in fitness. He kindly helped me review this book. (Noah at Priority Strength, http://prioritystrength.com. Check him out; dude's the real deal.) He wanted me to be sure you all knew that this "your knees shouldn't ever go beyond your toes in weight-bearing exercise" stuff is baloney. Feel free to internet the topic; it's well-discussed, so I'm not going to go there. I'm not saying "never put knees beyond toes." Per our discussion, that's baloney. In the context of this pose, we are just trying to make a shape that targets a particular area of the body.

OPTIONS

- ◆ Arm Variation: If crossing the wrists isn't available to you, just place your hands on your opposite shoulders like you're giving yourself a hug.

- ◆ To increase the strength work around your chest and shoulders, don't cross your arms at all. Just press your forearms together in front of your face and hold them there.

- ◆ Baby Eagle: To increase the challenge in Eagle, sit as low as you can into it. (The lower you go, the more your standing knee will shift forward. This is fine, as long as we keep the weight centered over the middle or middleback of the standing foot.) If you can, touch your bottom elbow to your bottom knee, round your spine, and tuck your chin to your chest.

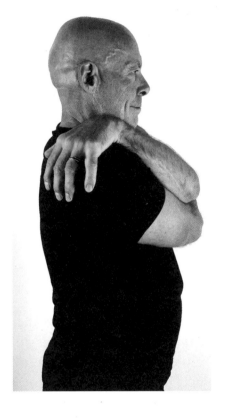

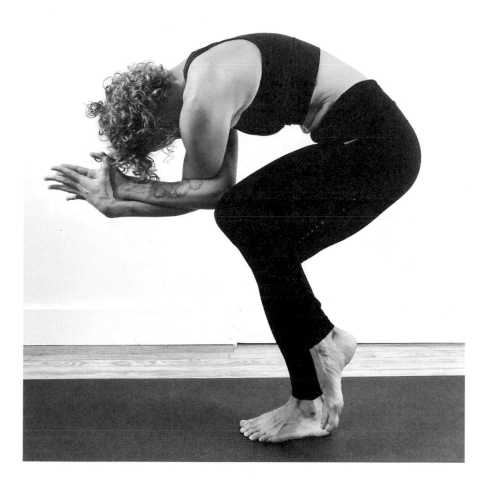

GOALS

- simultaneous opening of major joints (shoulders and hips) while strengthening upper back and glutes
- engagement of the kidney wings and back-body breathing
- stability in the standing ankle

Intermission: On Knee Locking

For a long time I taught a method that advocated knee-locking, where the knee is extended as far as it can go, usually under significant load. I've since come around. In Foundations, we don't lock the standing knee, particularly in balancing poses where nearly the entire weight of the body is on the joint.

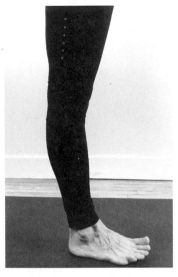

A mildly hyperextended knee. Summer's the closest we have to a hyperextender among our group of "models" and hers is fairly mild. However, you can get the idea; the line of the shin and the line of the femur are not the same. Her shin is leaning backward, driving the weight of the body back into the knee capsule.

The Cruciate Ligaments—Anterior and Posterior (ACL & PCL)—are the primary structures responsible for stabilizing the knee joint in extension, when the knee is locked. They're the things that stop your knee from buckling backwards.[71] They are a type of tissue called "articular ligaments." While ligaments are viscoelastic and can bounce back to their original shape after strain is released, if they are taken beyond a certain range, they can gradually become overstretched. Like a plastic bag that's been stretched out, ligaments that have been overstretched will not return to their original length.[72] If they're made longer, then that's pretty much their new length. (Also: ligaments are notoriously difficult to heal due to limited blood flow.)

---

[71] This is not their only job, to be clear, but it's a big part of their role in the body.

[72] https://benthamopen.com/contents/pdf/TOREHJ/TOREHJ-6-1.pdf

Your cruciate ligaments are super strong, largely because they do very important work in your body; they prevent your knees from buckling backward. However, there is no tissue in your body that will not deform given enough pressure for enough time, so it's important we refrain from placing undue pressure on connective tissue, particularly articular ligaments. Consider how much time a committed yoga student spends with the entire weight of their body on one leg, often with their center of gravity shifted forward beyond the hips.

This does not mean we should put *no* pressure on the ACL and PCL. Ligaments—like pretty much the rest of your body—are kept healthy through activity. They often respond positively to stress as long as it is not excessive. If the ACL and PCL become too long from excessive strain, a locked knee will likely begin to rest in hyperextension.

KNEE HYPEREXTENSION & POSTURE

Movement or structural issues are never strictly localized; they don't only affect one place in your body. Ask anyone who has had a major ankle sprain; they'll tell you they feel its effects in their whole leg and maybe elsewhere as well. Your body operates in a state of constant cooperation and communication. If one thing is out of whack, other stuff compensates. Maladaptations—problematic changes in the way you hold and move your body—reverberate throughout the system.

On the most basic level, the tissue that moves (or stabilizes) your knee directly influences the tissue that moves (or stabilizes) your pelvis. In some cases, like your major thigh muscles—the quads and hamstrings and adductors— they're the exact same tissue. So if you change the tension structure around your knee, you change the tension structure around your pelvis.

In my experience with knee locking, two common body patterns start to show up over time: Anterior Pelvic Tilt with pronounced low back compression and Posterior Pelvic Tilt with a significant shift of the hips forward over the toes. (Recall from earlier, the body patterns of kyphosis and swayback both likely include a degree of hyperextension in the knees.) When we lock the knee in standing positions, we run the risk of exacerbating maladaptive patterns in the low back, core muscles, hip flexors, shoulders, ankles, and neck. We also run the potential risk of creating these very patterns where they did not exist before.

SEXUAL DIMORPHISM[73] IS IN PLAY HERE, TOO

Women,[74] who make up the vast majority of yoga students, are potentially more susceptible to the issues of knee hyperextension for a couple reasons. Women are generally more flexible, potentially due in part to increased levels of the hormone Relaxin.[75] Also, women may have a greater tendency toward "quadriceps dominance," a muscle imbalance where the quads activate before the hamstrings when the foot lands during walking or running.[76]

Yoga in the west has, over decades, developed a popular image that is primarily bendy and female.[77] If you're bendy and female, yoga may be

---

[73] Sexual dimorphism is the difference in male and female morphology in plants and animals. In humans, sex is determined by gonads, sex hormones, internal reproductive organs, external genitalia, and the presence of a Y chromosome.

[74] The terms "woman" and "man" are used in this book to indicate male-bodied and female-bodied human beings, according to sexual dimorphism. Important to acknowledge that not everyone lives their lives according these terms, and there are intersex human beings, as well. Please forgive the linguistic shortcut, a full dive into this topic is beyond the scope of this here book.

[75] This is the hormone that allows female bodies to stretch beyond their "normal" limits during pregnancy, at which time Relaxin kinda floods the system. I swear to God that's its real name, I'm not making this up.

[76] Lephart, Scott, M.; Ferris, Cheryl, M.; Riemann, Bryan, L.; Myers, Joseph, B.; Fu, Freddie, H., "Gender Differences in Strength and Lower Extremity Kinematics During Landing," *Clinical Orthopaedics and Related Research* 401 (August 2002): 162-169. https://journals.lww.com/clinorthop/Fulltext/2002/08000/Gender_Differences _in_Strength_and_Lower_Extremity.19.aspx

[77] Don't believe me? At time of writing, just one of the last sixty-five issues of *Yoga Journal Magazine* featured a man on the cover. This is not a complaint, men don't necessarily need more representation. (Though I do wish more men would practice yoga, and this sort of begs the art-imitates-life/life-imitates-art question.) I'm just pointing out that our cultural image of yoga is predominantly female.

more appealing to you because you'll feel more comfortable and capable in the practice. The upshot of all of this is that flexible women are pretty much the core of the yoga market. So the population at increased risk of knee hyperextension (as well as other issues of hypermobility) is the same population most associated with yoga.

OK BUT SOME PEOPLE DO THIS KNEE-LOCKING THING VERY WELL

Hyperextension in the knees is not a universal concern. It is possible to create and maintain balanced strength in an upright leg during balancing poses. Human anatomy is diverse and variable. Certain bodies can do certain things with more stability than others. This isn't simply a matter of expertise. Bone structure, tension patterns, and general flexibility are major factors; I have seen hundreds of teachers and experienced students practice knee locking with excessive hyperextension.

Remember, Foundations is designed as an All Levels practice for groups, not a specialized program for proficient/well-suited individuals. It is designed to be accessible to and good for people of all body types. If I tell a group of people to lock their knees, some may be capable of doing it in a healthy way. Many may not.

THE REAL QUESTION: WHAT IS THE POINT?

So here's a question: even if knee-locking isn't bad, why do it? What is the benefit? While knee-locking can potentially promote balanced strength in the muscles of the thigh, so does practicing balancing postures with a slight bend in the knee.

In my experience, the main benefit is it lets you go deeper into some poses. Knee locking is a prime example of depth-seeking at the joint's end range of motion. You can go much further in Standing Bow, for example, if you sink the weight of the body into the back of the knee capsule. Of course, you get to choose if depth is your primary goal, but in Foundations we emphasize healthy neutral and repatterning over depth.

Big Toe Pose

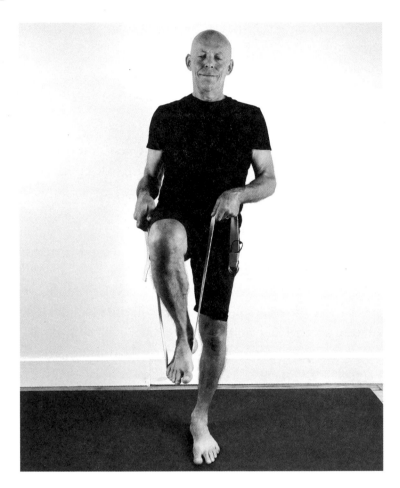

SETUP

Grab a yoga strap.[78] Start with your hands on your hips. Bend your knees a smidge and shift the weight to your left foot. Establish the contact of your left heel on the floor very strongly. Feel the connection between your heel and your hip. Imagine them as a deeply integrated, unified structure. This structure will keep you stable during the pose.

---

[78] If you don't have one, a belt or a towel or a bike chain will do just fine.

Lift your right knee up in the marching position, so it's about level with your hip. Take a moment to adjust your hips, so they're relatively level to the floor and relatively square to the front of the mat. Take a moment here with your chest upright and your heart open.

Place the strap under your right foot so it cradles the arch like a stirrup.

ENTRANCE

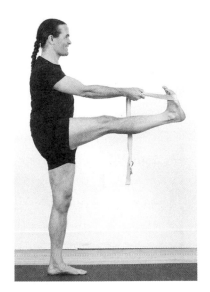

Inhale: Lift your chest up and stand tall.

Exhale: Steadily kick your leg forward until it is straight out in front of you. (If fully straight isn't available, just do what you can while maintaining upright, Healthy Neutral in the spine.)

ASSESSMENT

◆ Notice where the weight is traveling in the foot. It often likes to shift forward. Your toes may grip the mat; instead try to keep them dynamic and responsive.

◆ Maintain upright posture, even if it means you can't kick out all the way. Stand like you mean it, shoulders back and eyes steady.

BREATHING

In some ways this pose is simply the practice of standing up with extra challenge added. You might call it "Intense Standing-Up Pose." Your grounded leg, torso, and neck are all in a simple upright standing position. We have simply added the unusual challenge of lifting one leg toward horizontal.

Practice breathing in a way that supports an upright, stable posture. Imagine the inhale gently opening the kidney wings and collarbones. Exhale to stabilize the belly, especially at the seatbelt, and get tall. Keep your neck ungripped.

OPTIONS

If kicking out is not available to you for any reason, simply hold the strap and stay in the marching position.

If you don't have a strap, just put your right hand on your right knee and stand tall.

For advancement, you might experiment with releasing the strap and holding your leg out horizontally, without support. From this position, try pointing your toes and lifting your arms up straight over your head.

GOALS

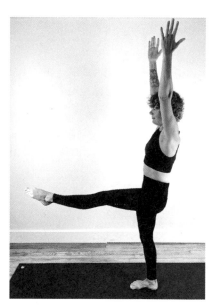

Advanced Big Toe Pose.

- ◆ establish Healthy Neutral in an upright standing position

- ◆ strengthen the back

- ◆ strengthen the standing leg and both hips

- ◆ open the hamstring of the lifted leg

- ◆ strengthen the hip flexors of the lifted leg (especially in the advanced position)

- ◆ decompress the spine

Revolved Big Toe Pose

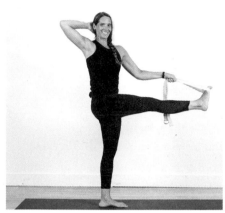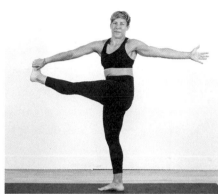

SETUP

Standing on the left leg, do Big Toe Pose with your right leg kicked forward. Depending on your body type and flexibility, you may be able to do this one without a strap.

ENTRANCE

Take hold of the strap—or your right foot, if you're not using the strap—with your left hand. Stay upright in your torso.

Place the palm of your right hand on the back of your skull, then turn your right elbow back until your heart center starts to turn right.

ASSESSMENT

As in all of our balancing work, notice how you're distributing the weight of your body through your foot. We want to keep the heel heavy and the toes soft. Notice if you're rolling inside or outside on the foot.

There's no need to try to crank this twist; just turn your right shoulder back and open your heart. Overall, the shape of the posture is not very complex, though it can be challenging. We want to focus on simply setting the tension pattern and allowing the breath to move.

EVERY BREATH IS A REP

Imagine you're at the gym lifting weights. (I know, that may not be your cup of tea. For some of you I might as well ask you to imagine doing your taxes. I get it; just roll with me for a hot minute.) Each time you perform a set action—moving some object or body part in a certain cycle, first one way then back the other— you're doing a "repetition" or "rep." The whole point of reps is the development of a body pattern—usually a strength pattern, but not always—that reinforces whatever action you're performing.[79] With standard reps, the pattern could be described as *action, return, action, return, action, return.* If you do a bench press, the *action* happens every time you push the bar up. The *return* is the lowering of the bar to your chest.

That was really pedantic; I'm sorry. We're going to the very basics here, breaking apart what a "rep" means, because this concept applies directly to your yoga practice, and your body patterns. It's important to remember that breathing is a muscular action. It requires power to create movement to create a pressure differential to pump air in and out of the lungs. You move your body in some way, then return to stasis. This is usually, though not always, performed as: *inhale-action, exhale-return,* in which the inhale is the "lift."

Over the course of a day, you will perform around twenty thousand breaths. You are, in a way, doing very light weightlifting all day, every day. In a way, every breath you take is a form of muscular development, a kind of ongoing practice. In fact, it's the most important muscular practice over which you have voluntary control.[80]

---

[79] Turns out the debate about "low reps" (few reps at high weight) and "high reps" (lots of reps at lower weight) is a fairly energetic one among people who do such things. I'll not dive into those weeds, for there be dragons, and those dragons drink protein shakes and are not to be messed with.

[80] Gotta throw one up here in respect for the amazing work of the cardiac muscles, the true champions in the world of muscle activity. Underappreciated because they're involuntary and internal, these muscles are truly the stars of the myofascial system. Myocardium, endocardium, epicardium, we see you even though we can't see you. Thanks, heart. You're great. Love you.

When we assume unusual body positions in yoga, we change the shape of the breath. That is, we change the way in which our muscular system activates to get that ever-essential *action-return, action-return*. Every pose puts different demands on different tension patterns. For example, in a twist, your abdominal muscles are, at the very least, subject to unusual tension patterns, your respiratory diaphragm will probably not drop as easily as normal, and the tension across your chest will be asymmetrical. One side of your rib cage will move differently from the other. You'll have to use a different strength pattern, a different organization of muscles, to take a full breath. The *action-return* will activate an unusual pattern.

You can take this idea and extend it, explore it, and use it to inform your practice. Forward fold? Breathe one way. Back bend? Breathe another. Front side compression? You get the idea. You're taking your breath to the gym, making it do different exercises, forming it and shaping it and making it stronger. Yoga poses are unique and powerful ways to influence your movement by patterning the strength and motion of your breath.

BREATHING

Normal, full breaths are fine here. You may find it helpful to breathe into the right side of your chest, to release the pectoral muscles and unlock your shoulder a bit.

To explore further, imagine the inhale moving from your left hip, up past your navel, to your right shoulder. Then move the exhale from your right shoulder, down your back, to your left hip. Explore this loop from hip to shoulder and see if it helps you open the twist more comfortably.

OPTIONS

If kicking out isn't working for you, simply perform the revolve in the marching position.

Like in Big Toe, you can make this one more challenging by dropping your strap, foot, or knee from your left hand. Spread your arms wide and try to keep your right leg horizontal as you open the twist. If you can hold it, make sure you're breathing. Doesn't count if you ain't breathing.

GOALS

- pattern Healthy Neutral in upright rotation
- develop core stability
- strengthen the standing leg and both hips

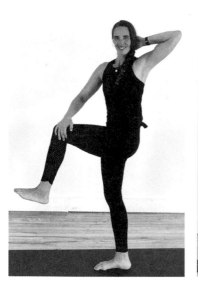
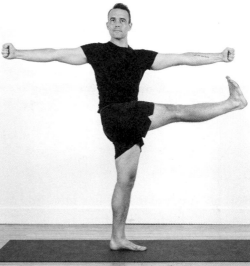

Core Strength Quad Stretch

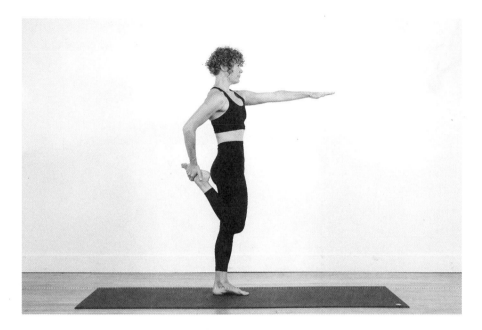

SETUP

1. From standing with your hands on your hips, step your right foot back behind you a bit. Curl your toes underneath so they're pointing to the back of your mat. Take a moment here to stretch the front of your foot and ankle.

2. Reach your right arm up and lean slightly to the left. Take a breath and feel for a long stretch from your right thigh to your right shoulder.

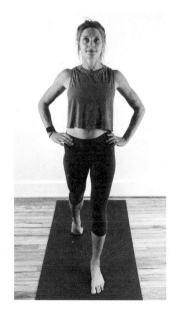

3. Slowly bend your right knee and lift your foot toward your butt.
(Don't reach back and grab your foot, yet. Just try to pull your heel
as close to your hips as possible. With any luck your hamstrings
are firing like crazy now. Good. If they're cramping up, take a deep
breath. Feel free to curse my name.[81])

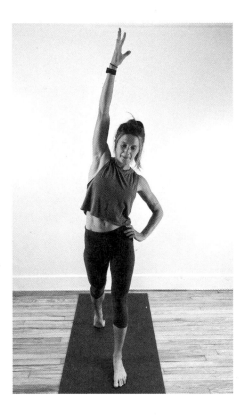 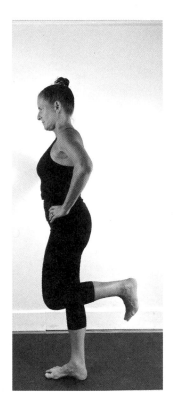

---

[81] Quick reminder: my name is Kyle. So it'd be something like, "May malevolent
guardians of unforgiving shadow realms bring Kyle wasteful harvests and the scorn
of his beloveds, until the sky turns to dust at the end of days." Or whatever. Come
up with your own; it's an opportunity to be creative.

ENTRANCE

Take hold of the outside of your right foot with your right hand. Extend your left arm straight ahead with your fingers together. Gently bend your right elbow as you draw your belly in strongly.

ASSESSMENT

We call this "core strength quad stretch" because it is both of those things, and core strength goes first. There's a tendency to try to make the quad stretch portion of this primary and add the core strength on top. Unfortunately, that's a good way to lose the pose entirely. If the

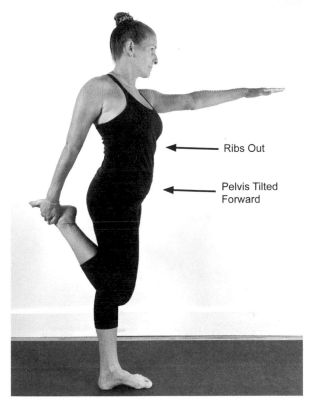

Ribs Out

Pelvis Tilted
Forward

It's very common for students to do the quad stretch by simply drawing the knee back and down, so they tilt the pelvis forward and drive the ribs out.

pelvis, abdomen, and lower back aren't stabilized before we apply leverage, it will be difficult to stabilize them later on. So, before you start to pull on your foot with any real power, take a moment to run a quick checklist:

- ribs in
- tail down
- seatbelt on

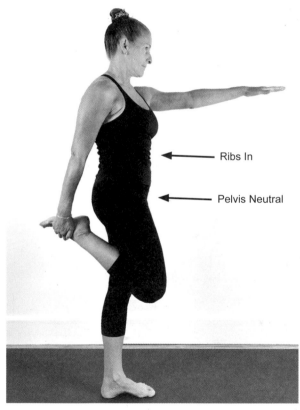

Ribs In

Pelvis Neutral

Stabilize the spine first. Hold the ribs in and the tail down, then begin to gently activate the quad stretch. Your knee will probably not go as far back, but that's fine.

TIDAL VOLUME, RESERVE VOLUME, AND CORE STRENGTH

One way to empower your exhales is to truly explore their full depth. In a normal inhale-exhale cycle, you use what is called your tidal volume, the amount of air you turn over with a normal, unforced breath. Then you have something called your reserve volume, which is how much air you can *make yourself* inhale or exhale. Your biggest exhale possible is your exhale tidal volume (ETV) + exhale reserve volume (ERV). (Don't worry, there's no math here. Unless you *want* math. In which case, go calculate the surface area of your nearest rhombus.)

So try this out: Take a normal breath. Just in and out, no big deal. Now take the biggest inhale you can without popping. Full lung capacity. Now exhale as much air as possible. Empty out as completely as you can.[82] I'll ask you to notice the difference in effort between a full reserve inhale and a full reserve exhale; the inhale is certainly work, but a complete exhale? That's annoyingly, distractingly difficult.

In order to perform the kind of exhale we're talking about here, you have to powerfully engage deep core muscles. Your abs and back and pelvic floor all have to get in the game in some way. You might find that as you perform this complete exhale your core muscles are tightening up around your spine like a corset. See, your "full exhale" muscles are also your "spinal support" muscles. Healthy breathing and healthy spines are fundamentally interconnected. As you practice, I invite you to experiment with this idea; you can help create spinal stability and core strength through intentional breathing. The occasional practice of complete exhales is one way to actively participate in this process.

---

[82] You will not physically be able to get *all* the air out of your lungs. If your lungs actually "emptied" they would collapse, which is not something your body would allow to happen, and is also clearly unsound yoga practice.

BREATHING

Use your exhales to tone the abdomen and support the spine. See if your inhales can make you taller without back-bending.

You will likely discover that at the bottom of full exhales, you feel a more powerful stretch in the quads. Part of what's happening there is that your abdominal muscles are contracting to drive air out, which pulls the front of your pelvis upward, which draws the tops of the quads upward as well (because they insert onto the front of the pelvis), which lengthens them inside the pose.

Another way of saying this is, your quads are essentially integrated with your breath, so, in a way, your legs breathe. In this position, that breath stretches your quads. Behold, my friend, the Josephine that is your miraculous body.

OPTIONS

If holding your foot behind you isn't available here, try hooking your foot in a strap and using that to create the "hold."

If balance is tough for you, put a hand on a wall for added support.

GOALS

- ◆ stabilize the core muscles
- ◆ lengthen the quads of the lifted leg
- ◆ pattern Healthy Neutral in upright posture

Standing Bow

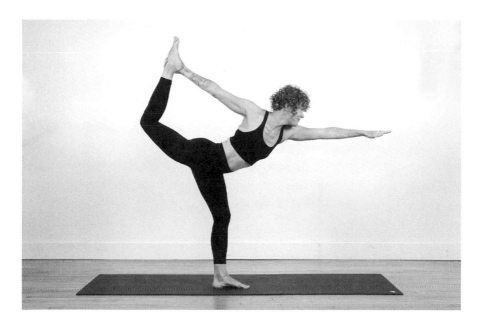

SETUP

From Core Strength Quad Stretch, run your right palm up and over your toes to take a grip on the inner arch of the foot. (Note: this should "open" your shoulder, turning your bicep outward and your elbow back.)

Square your hips forward.

Lift your left arm high. Get tall.

ENTRANCE

Inhale: Lift your heart and reach up to the ceiling.

Exhale: Steadily lean forward and start to gently kick into your right hand.

Take your time coming down. If you rush or overexert yourself, you will likely "spin out" and tilt your right hip out of line with your left. In my experience, this is the most common issue for students, particularly if they're overinvested in chasing depth or "impressive" poses. Keep in mind that the entrances, or transitions, are often where we get off track. Things get a little wonky when we're in motion, especially when we're balancing on one leg. Take your time and sweat the details.

ASSESSMENT

The primary goals of Standing Bow are: standing hip (and leg) strength and integration, right shoulder and chest opening, and spinal extension (back bend). As long as your hips are relatively level and you're not locking your knee, you'll get the first one pretty well. Spinal extension will come in time, usually from depth developed in other postures like Camel.

The shoulder (and chest) opening part is important to remember, because it can go far toward reorganizing how we hold tension in the pose. It can help to reduce the intensity of the "kick" action in the pose, at least at the start, so we don't add too much work to the shape in the process of setting it up. This is something to keep in mind setting up all balancing poses. In a balancing pose, your body is often a fair degree closer to "emergency mode" with regard to keeping you vertical and not, you know, turning into a puddle on the floor. With one point of support instead of two, the chances of falling over are greater. As a result, you're more likely to use your habitual tension patterns because they're better established and more stable.

All this is to say, go slowly and don't overemphasize depth. If you aren't well integrated through your standing leg and hips, we'll miss the good work there, as well as in the hips and core. I'll warn you now: the resulting pose will not look as cool on Instagram. It will get you fewer clicks, because it doesn't arrive at a glorious standing split. That's OK. Put the big picture over big postures. Let's make that a rule, actually. Rule 5: Big Picture Over Big Postures.

ON TECHNOLOGY, IMAGERY, AND YOGA PRACTICE

Over the last seventy years or so, the world of personal photography has grown by leaps and bounds, and it's exploded in the last decade with the development of cell phones with digital cameras. We are living in a world of pictures, with visual stimulus cascading into our brains. Handheld access to a near infinite constellation of content is overwhelming, and it warps our brains. The way we construct an idea of "normal" or "good" in nearly every aspect of our lives has almost instantly transformed as a digital monsoon has made landfall on our psychological shores. An image of B. K. S. Iyengar doing a Standing Bow pose in *Light on Yoga* was once remarkable. Now it's barely worth noticing. I see that stuff all day on Facebook.

At the same time, yoga developed into a professional pursuit across the globe. There are currently six thousand–plus yoga studios in the United States alone. In a way, this is awesome. It's also created some challenges. As competition among studios has increased, studio owners have turned to teacher trainings as a way to generate revenue. Certifications are, for many studios, a major source of income. So the yoga teaching pool is heavily saturated. Everyone and their cousin seems to have a two-hundred-hour certification these days, and there is market pressure for yoga teachers to stand out in an increasingly competitive environment. This need to stand out in the internet era has created a sort of arms race for our attention, particularly online. To meet this demand, yoga teachers (and yoga models) often resort to contortionism and glamour shots, and sometimes both. We collectively create imagery that is more and more extreme each day and broadcast it to the community at large.[83]

Much in the same way that the projected lives of friends and strangers on social media warps our understanding of happiness, these projected images of yoga poses can warp our understanding of bodies. If a young,

---

[83] There is another concern in this realm: the hypersexualization of yoga online. I will leave that for more qualified thinkers than I to address in full. But needless to say, I'm concerned.

lean, fit, smiling person with perfect skin and a *mala* necklace performs an extreme back bend on Instagram, and that picture gets thousands of likes, we notice that.[84] That image, and the social validation it receives, forms our opinions about what we should pursue. Even if the image or post is not explicitly advocating this extreme pose, its mere presentation in a positive light affects us.[85]

What we get from this arms race is a cultural attitude about yoga poses and healthy bodies that often idealizes contortionism. It's important for us to repeatedly ask ourselves, how am I measuring value? What are my physical goals? If we are mindful about these questions and the way we answer them, we are less likely to pursue practices that may not fit our personal needs.

Oh, one more thing. Regardless of how you choose to practice, and who you choose to learn from, consider for a moment the interconnectedness of this holistic system. In this society at least, popularity has the power to override efficacy; financial realities define the practice that shows up in the yoga room. You might imagine a sort of Josephine in all of this. The practice is in the studio, which is in the economy. They are components and they are all one.

---

[84] I have done all these things. I am not immune.

[85] One of the things the ad men understand that eludes many of the rest of us is that images influence our beliefs and behavior even *when we consciously reject them.* There's not really a "don't create meaning out of this information" setting in the human brain. It's always trying to interpret sensory data—especially visual information like pictures—even if it's doing it unconsciously. These things matter to us, even when we think they don't.

BREATHING

Explore the capacity of an inhale to open the right shoulder (the arm reaching back to hold the foot.) The pectoral muscles can often respond well to this intention, as they can gently open with the pulse of the breath.

Use your exhales to stabilize the lower ribs in particular. When we're doing heart openers or back bends, it's important to keep in mind the tendency of the rib cage to flare out and compress the mid-back. The exhales in particular allow the opportunity to integrate the core muscles and hold the spine stable.

If you are looking to get a little funky with it, think about the breath moving in, around, and through the left hip (standing leg). Notice how the movement of full breath may affect this structure, the fulcrum of the pose.

OPTIONS

If you are having difficulty holding your foot in your hand, use a strap to close the distance.

It's not uncommon for the hips to spin out when the right shoulder is drawn back by the kicking leg. To help turn your heart forward, opening the chest more, place your left palm on the back of your head and open your elbow out wide so it's pointing straight away from your ear. This will increase the tension across the top of your chest and begin to draw the heart center back toward the front plane.

If balance is a challenge, feel free to do this next to a wall.

GOALS

- open the left chest and shoulder
- pattern stability and balance into the right hip
- pattern stability in rotation during spinal extension

Airplane

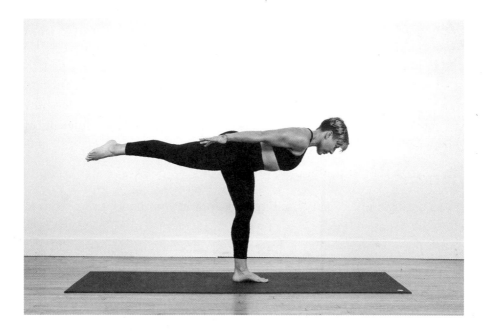

SETUP

This one goes in phases so we can establish some fundamentals:

1. Take your arms overhead and step your right foot back. Rock your weight into your left heel, then lift your right foot an inch off the ground. Keep a healthy bend in your left leg, knee stacked over your ankle.

2. Sweep your arms down by your sides, like an airplane, and draw your ribs in. Line up your torso with your back leg.

At the end of your setup, we want to have a straight line from your head to your right foot. Notice if you've got your head forward of your shoulders or your mid-back compressed in a back bend. Try to keep your ribs in and your ears over your shoulders.

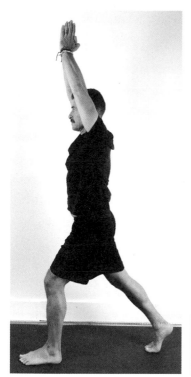
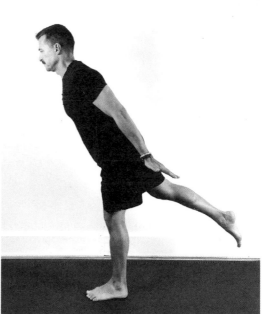

What we're setting up is a Healthy Neutral position, like in standing, except we're about to make that line horizontal instead of vertical.

ENTRANCE

Keeping your hips square (ish), slowly bring yourself down toward horizontal. Imagine you have something straight and rigid, like a board or a dust mop, on your back, and try to hold it along this line: back of the skull–between shoulder blades–glutes–right heel.

ASSESSMENT

Like in Standing Bow, it's very common for the hips to "spin out" on this one. Your right hip might lift up well above the level of your left. What's probably happening here is your left hip doesn't want to do the work. It's trying to cheat. If the pelvis is tilted diagonally, your glutes in particular don't have to work as hard (and most of us these days have cheater glutes).

There's some simple physics involved here. Holding a weight straight out on a horizontal plane requires more force than holding it on a diagonal. You can test this out. Hold something like a small pig or a Vitamix out straight to the side, with your arm level. Notice how difficult that is. Now hold it up at a 45-degree angle. It's harder horizontal, right? That's happening with your hips in Airplane Pose too. If you lift your right hip up on a diagonal, it takes less force to keep it stable than with your hips level.[86]

---

[86] Disclaimer: There is other stuff going on here, like which muscle groups and fibers you are using. But the principle is in play regardless.

EXPLORATION: WHERE IS BALANCE, AND HOW?

If you're challenged by one-legged postures, you might explore reorienting your focus. I find that students who have trouble with balance often focus almost exclusively on their feet and the floor. But your feet and ankles are not the most important balancing points; your hips are. Keep in mind that during all balancing poses, the standing hip is the fulcrum of the body. It is close to the center of gravity, has a wide range of mobility and complex musculature, and serves as the "meeting point" between the stable foundation—the leg—and the balancing mass—the rest of your body. Energy and strength move through that one major joint. If we have power and control there, we can balance more easily. Keep steady focus on your hips and you'll likely discover your balancing practice improves almost immediately.

Or: Just Trust Your Body

There is some interesting evidence that humans are actually *worse* at balancing when they think about balancing.[87] Try this: Get your cell phone. Go into Airplane Pose, then compose a long text or internet message to your favorite middle school teacher telling them how much they helped you during a weird time because, I mean, come on, eighth grade is the worst.

Go try it now. Seriously, real quick. It'll take you one minute.

Totally waiting ...

OK, you back? How was your balance when you did that? Did you feel anything? If you need to go back and try it again, go for it. Everybody's different, but for most people the external task—composing a text message—increases their stability. The interesting thing is that we don't really *notice* our balance has improved because, you know, we aren't paying attention. (Oh, also: send that text now. Seriously, make someone's day.)

If you're falling over and you try consciously to rebalance yourself, there are decent odds you will overcompensate and worsen the situation. Our thoughts themselves are not super great at balance because balance happens pre-thought; your body makes adjustments faster than your conscious mind. So it's arguably best to leave the lion's share of work of balance to your instinctive internal systems. In yoga, the gaze is often prioritized to maintain balance. This practice distracts your conscious attention. You stop thinking about balance quite as much when you meditate on a specific visual point.[88]

---

[87] Nancy H. McNevin and Gabriele Wulf, "Attentional Focus on Supra-postural Tasks Affects Postural Control," *Human Movement Science* 21:2 (2002): 187–202, doi:10.1016/S0167-9457(02)00095-7.

[88] This is not the only reason this practice helps with balance, but it is potentially part of the benefit.

Every now and then, after you've built a balancing pose with a well-structured pattern, try thinking about something else. Think about ... gardening. Or the benefits of a circular waste model in home construction. Or the astonishing accomplishment that is Peter Jackson's film adaptation of J. R. R. Tolkien's Lord of the Rings trilogy. (But nothing else. Those are your only options of things to think about.)

Hold your shoulders in line with the body, not hunched forward. This may require a bit of focus as you work to hold the shoulder blades on your back. If this is a challenge in the beginning, just keep at it. We are working to make your upper back strong, particularly the rhomboid muscles that draw your shoulder blades together. This will help improve your standing posture, as a strong upper back will help you correct or avoid shoulder hunch.

Take special care with the position of your skull as well. Often when the body moves toward horizontal, people jut their heads forward and hang the weight of the head at the back of the neck. Doing your best to keep the ears in line with the shoulders, just like in healthy upright standing, slowly approach horizontal. This may require a good deal of effort, particularly if forward head carriage is a major concern for you. Take your time. The muscles that resist forward head carriage are often underdeveloped and need repeated training to restore their proper strength. Don't push too hard; we don't want you to tighten up and struggle.

RAMP THE NECK

Slightly drop the chin and take the jawline back toward the neck. This should make the back of the neck long. If you take it all the way, it looks sort of like "military neck." You might feel the muscles in the front of the neck turning on strongly here; relish it. Those muscles are the ones that help hold your head upright, so you don't drop into forward head carriage. If we make them strong, we are doing great work in service of healthy human posture.[89]

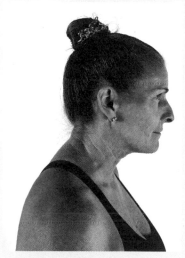

Forward head carriage.

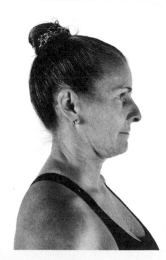

Ramped neck.

---

[89] Credit where it's due: I picked up this concept from Katy Bowman, who is a wonderful teacher and bodyworker. I highly recommend her books, podcast, and blog to anyone interested in exploring human movement. She is more of a "natural movement" person than a yoga person, which I actually really dig since she brings a fresh perspective for teachers and students of yoga.

BREATHING

With the torso in Healthy Neutral, ribs in and shoulders back, try to take full breaths without letting your abdominal muscles disengage. Think about the wave of breath moving in your back just as fully as the front body. Use your exhales to stabilize your core and draw the ribs in.

If full breaths are difficult at first, go slowly. Make sure your breathing is not causing you to grip around the shoulders and neck. Despite its relatively simple shape, Airplane Pose puts a lot of demand on the body. Especially when it's done with proper alignment. Do what is available to you while you maintain comfortable, mindful breathing.

OPTIONS

If you're particularly invested in stabilizing your core and avoiding the "drop" into a back bend, point your arms at the floor. This will reduce the strength needed to hold you in the position. Also, with your arms in the front plane—pointing the same way as your heart—you clear some space in the mid-back, and it's easier to knit the ribs. You might try setting up the pose this way and slowly bring the arms back over the duration of the posture.

If it's not available for you to get horizontal while holding Healthy Neutral, prioritize Healthy Neutral. Bring yourself down to whatever angle you can while maintaining the stability of the pose around your torso and spine.

GOALS

- ◆ pattern strength and balance into left hip
- ◆ pattern Healthy Neutral under increased challenge or at horizontal
- ◆ strengthen glutes, hamstrings of the lifted leg
- ◆ strengthen the upper back

Revolved Half Moon

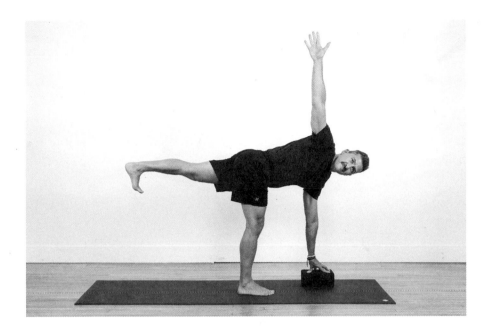

SETUP

From Airplane, drop your hands to the floor. Keep your back leg up.

Set a yoga block under your right hand.

The Decker Pulse

Named after the teacher who implemented it into Foundations, a physical therapist named Emily Decker, this "pulse" is a kind of reset between Airplane and the Revolved Half Moon. We use it to ensure the core is engaged and the glutes are activated before twisting the spine.

It goes like this:

1. **Inhale:** Lift your chin up and look forward.

2. **Exhale:** Bend both knees and round your spine. Try to touch your forehead to your knees.

3. Gently kick your right foot (the lifted foot) out to the right, away from the midline. This internally rotates your right femur and helps activate your right glutes.

4. Keeping the right foot pointing out like this, inhale and slowly extend your right leg as you lift your torso out of the rounded position.

The stability of the entire structure moves through the hips, so take special care to engage the glutes throughout, even after the leg is extended.

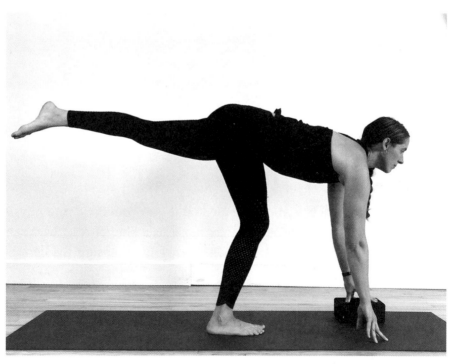

Decker Pulse, step 1 (by the way, the model here is the actual human being Emily Decker. Totally not a fictional character, but a corporeal person who is generous and kind and frighteningly smart.)

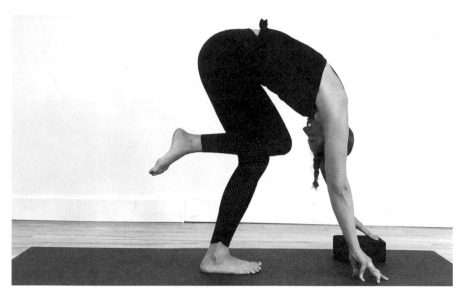

Decker Pulse, step 2.

Once you've done your pulse, press your right hand down strongly on the block. Place your left hand in the Stamos position, where your palm is on the back of your head. Gently turn your left elbow up toward the ceiling, opening your chest to the left.

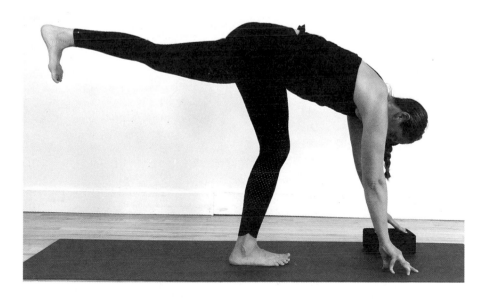

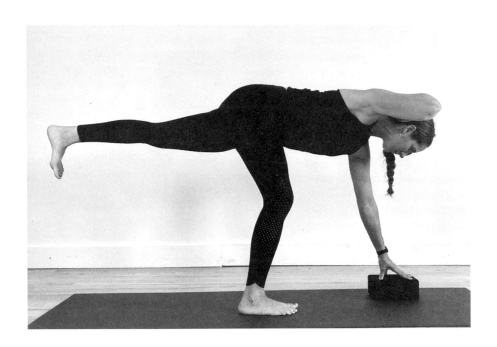

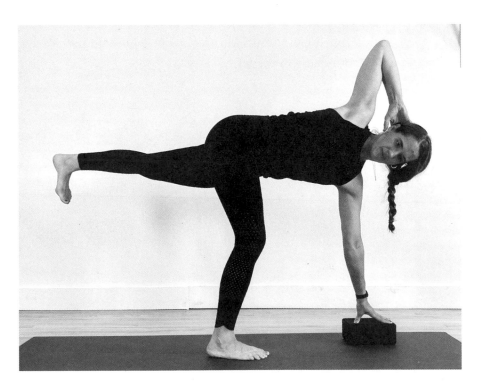

THE STAMOS

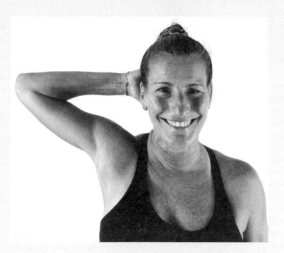

The Stamos is named after teen idol, *Full House* alum, and all-around dreamboat John Stamos. The idea is that when you put your hand behind your head and turn to the side like this, you resemble (you are?) someone with fantastic hair posing for a glamour shot.

Like many cultural norms, what started as a stupid joke grew beyond control into an actual term of use in a yoga community, and it has now shown up in an actual book for actual readers. I am now inviting you into this stupid joke and gleefully encourage you to use "the Stamos" as the proper name for this action.[90] I have yet to find another term for it, so let's just stick this flag into the moon and call it a day, shall we?

We perform the Stamos in twisting or revolving poses because it prevents cheating disguised as depth. It's pretty common that people try to

---

[90] One fantasy I have is that this usage normalizes and eventually people lose sight of the term's origin. Then someday some very sincere and dedicated yoga students try to figure out what "Stamos" means and find their way into the dusty recesses of the Library of Athens and seemingly "discover" a semi-rational, austere justification for the name, like, "*stamos* (archaic, verb). To empower by means of wagonry or seduction." I feel like we could do this.

"complete" a twist by tossing an arm toward the ceiling and calling it a day. But this doesn't really require spinal rotation; it just takes shoulder mobility. So, we can get the wrong idea that we are at some kind of "full expression" of the pose when we might just be twisting up our shoulder.

The Stamos prevents this cheat. It also helps develop upper back strength and opening across the chest, which are both important to counteracting shoulder hunch.

It should be noted that shoulders are complicated joints. For some people, this position doesn't really work. If you feel discomfort or pain, try putting your hand on your sacrum (at the small of your back) instead of behind your head.

ASSESSMENT

- Keep your back foot lifted. In fact, lift it as high as you can while maintaining the twist. If you're really looking to gain strength in your glutes, straightening and lifting the back leg is the most direct route during this pose.

- Make sure you're not gripping the back of your neck to look upward in the twist.

- Notice the tendency for the weight of the body to drift forward, placing the load of the posture in the front of the knee.

- Ungrip your toes from the floor. There's no need to lift them up or anything; we want proprioception—the tactile feedback of your toes against the floor—but notice if you're "grabbing" the ground with them.

- Keeping your back leg lifted, drive your hand down firmly into the floor. Try to establish a mental connection between your grounded hand and your grounded foot, moving through the arm, the torso, and the leg. This is a closed chain of contact that will stabilize you and help recruit your core strength in the pose.

BREATHING

The key here is to breathe evenly. This one is pretty hard when we're really dialed in, so don't overwork or tighten around your breath. Soften your jaw and use your exhales to stabilize the core in the twist.

If you like, this is an opportunity to explore full reserve-volume exhales: get as much air out as possible to stabilize and strengthen the core inside the rotation.

OPTIONS

◆ A block under your right (grounded) hand is a great option here. I actually consider it less of an "option" and more of a "must for beginners." Getting your torso level to the floor is much more important to the structure of the posture than doing it without props. We want to create a nice even, level line from the left heel to the crown of the head.

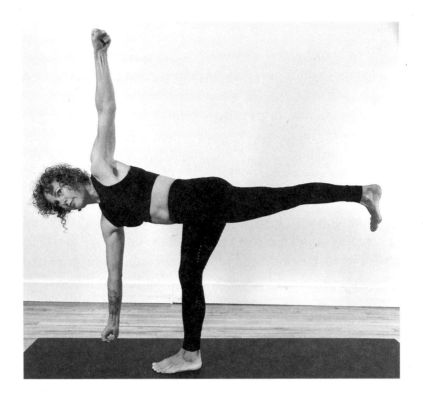

- ◆ If you are feeling very stable through the hips and can keep the back leg lifted, you can try the intermediate variation of the posture; float your right hand off the ground so you're now balancing the twist on just the left leg. If this works for you, next make both hands into fists and "punch" them both away from the heart. Feel how this strong action in the hands engages the arms and can give you more power to open the line across the heart.

GOALS

- ◆ open the left side chest while stabilizing and strengthening the upper back
- ◆ pattern toward Healthy Neutral in a horizontal rotation
- ◆ strengthen hips, particularly the glutes of the lifted leg
- ◆ develop core stability and balance

Separate Leg Sequence

Wide-Legged Dog

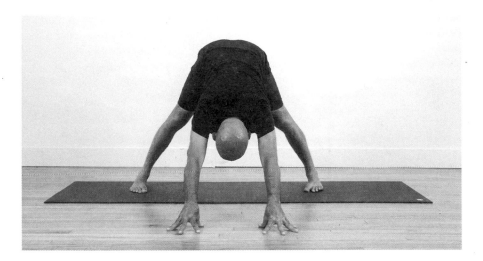

SETUP

Take a wide stance on your mat and bring your arms out wide, straight and level with the ground.

Inhale: Lift your heart.

Exhale: Bend your knees slightly and slowly descend, heart-first, toward the floor. As you reach the bottom of your capacity, let your hands drop to the ground.

Once you've reached the ground, take a moment to shift your body side to side, loosening the hips, ankles, and knees. Go easy, and move only as it feels comfortable for you.

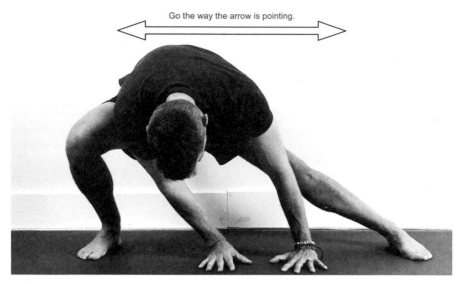

Go the way the arrow is pointing.

Side to sides. Let it move easily back and forth, to a depth that works for you.

Tent your fingertips on the floor and lift your torso up away from the floor, until you're touching the ground with your arms straight.

Take a moment here to establish Healthy Neutral in the spine. If you're stiffer, you will likely find your lower back is rounding into a hunched position. In this case, you've found the beginning of your pose; from here just work on gently arching your back until you reach Healthy Neutral.

ENTRANCE

If you are able to set your spine in Healthy Neutral, begin to walk your hands forward (the way your toes are pointing, basically). Without letting your hips move forward beyond your toes, walk those hands forward as far as you can while maintaining Healthy Neutral. If your spine starts to round forward, stop there and reestablish the position.

If it's available, walk your arms forward until your biceps are lined up by your ears. You may end up with a straight line from your wrists to your hips. You may not. Be sensitive with your shoulders and hamstrings.

ASSESSMENT

♦ If you're quite bendy, you may actually find yourself sinking into a back bend here. A normal lumbar curve is great, but occasionally the weight of the spine sinks into a deeper, unsupported position. If that is the case, draw your ribs in strongly until your core is engaged in support of Healthy Neutral. Exhales will help.

♦ Notice your toes; ungrip them if they're grabbing the floor.

♦ Imagine that your legs are straws, and the floor is a green vegan choco-nut smoothie with too much peanut butter. Try to "pull" the floor up to your hips through your legs. You may notice your legs tone and your hips stabilize.

♦ Avoid straightening your knees all the way for the duration of the pose. It may be helpful to spend a few breaths with the knees at their full range of motion, to open the posterior chain, but then bend them again to reengage the thigh muscles.

♦ Notice how you're carrying weight in your feet. Anchor the balls of the feet firmly and spread your toes to engage the muscles throughout your feet and ankles. Without shifting too much weight back into the heels, think about driving them down and back through the mat.

♦ **Josephine:** When you're working on your heels driving back, pay attention to the feelings in your hips. You might find the pelvis begins to tilt forward, lengthening your hamstrings.

♦ With your mind's eye, find the tops of your inner thighs. Think about spinning them back (the way your heels are pointing) internally rotating your thigh bones. Notice how this may create space in the back of the hips. If you feel the spin activating, tone your belly strongly and take deep breaths all the way down to the tailbone.

BREATHING

Easy peasy, from the sinuses to the hips. If you're in a back bend, use the exhale to stabilize the ribs back toward the spine.

This one is also an opportunity to explore full reserve-volume exhales.

OPTIONS

- If getting your hands to the floor in the beginning of the pose is not available to you, find some support. A yoga block (or seven) is a great option. We don't want you just hanging your upper body down without support. Once you have your hands planted on something stable, you are no longer in an open chain position and can recruit greater strength to stabilize your forward bend, and modify your pelvic position.

- If you reach full extension, with the torso lengthened forward in Healthy Neutral and the arms generally in line with the spine, then tone your belly strongly and experiment with lifting your hands off the floor. Be gentle. If this doesn't put too much pressure on your lower back, try turning your palms up like you're holding two bowls and gently lifting the bowls off the floor. You might explore bringing your torso and arms up until you're parallel to the floor.

This is a difficult option that requires a great deal of core strength. Don't rush it, as it can be trouble for your lower back if you try to go too far, too fast.

GOALS

- open the posterior chain through the hips and legs
- develop stability through the hips
- pattern Healthy Neutral into the torso

Vitruvian Person

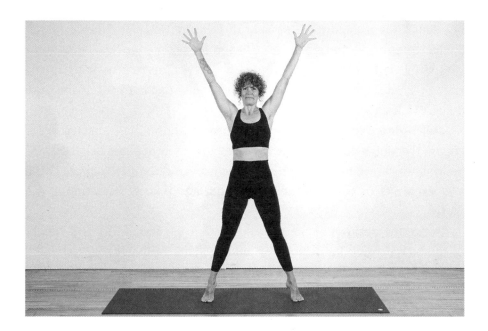

SETUP

Lift up from the ground and close your stance about a foot or so. Your feet should be wider than hip width, but not quite a full wide-legged position.

Place your hands on your hips, with your thumbs hooked over your glutes.

ENTRANCE

Rock back into your heels for a moment, then rock into the balls of your feet and start to lift your heels up. Come up high on your toes, as high as possible.

Dig your thumbs down onto your glutes to encourage your pelvis to stay tucked down underneath your heart.

If you can get up high on your toes and remain stable, you may extend your arms straight overhead.

ASSESSMENT

Vitruvian Person is in many ways upright standing practice. We're training your body to hold itself upright in Healthy Neutral with the added challenge of being up on your toes. Keep focus on your hips, especially. Notice the tendency toward tilting the pelvis forward as your quads engage. Mindfully establish neutral in the pelvis, so the load of the pose doesn't sink into the lower back.

Josephine: Notice how stabilizing your abdominal muscles helps engage the glutes. The abs in the front will lift the front of the pelvis toward neutral, which will force your glutes to activate as a counterbalance. These are two pieces of a whole: the abs balance and inform the action of the glutes.[91]

Notice the position of the ankles. It is not uncommon for the weight of the body to sink into the outer ankles. Many of us have lost stability and healthy tension in the outer ankle because of things like shoes and flat floors; in our day-to-day lives we often don't have to counteract the outward "roll" of weight in the ankle, so we may not have stable tension there.[92] If this is the case, when you go up on your toes you may "sink" the load of the posture outward, buckling the ankles away from each other. Take your time with this and mindfully correct the position. Try to line the bones of the foot with the tibia, your shin bone, so the line of force from your knees to your toes is relatively direct. This will take time and intention; don't rush it. Stabilizing your outer ankles will help make your knees healthy.

Try this: Imagine you've got a baby hippopotamus between your thighs. Give it a hug. Feel your adductors engage and take a deep breath. Remember that your adductors are rooted to your pelvis. They help stabilize the bottom of your spine. If we can get them to turn on effectively, they will help keep you balanced.

---

[91] And the QLs, and the diaphragm, and the quads, and …

[92] Imagine for a moment walking in the woods. If you step on a rock, you may tilt your ankle inward or outward. If you've not practiced counteracting this roll, over and over, your ankles may have lost some of their natural ability to do so.

JOSEPHINE: FEET, ANKLES, AND KNEES

Some of the muscles that help hold your outer ankle stable are the same muscles that help hold your outer knee stable. They integrate into the ligaments that keep your knee from buckling outward. The movement and stability of your foot is not just connected to the movement and stability of your knee; they are in some important ways the very same thing.

The peroneus longus muscle is particularly interesting in this regard. This slim muscle runs from the head of your fibula down the outside of your shin and inserts into a tendon that helps move your pinky toe and evert your foot.[93] In the world of shoes and flat floors, this muscle doesn't get much good work. Many modern humans have a hard time even moving their pinky toes, because they've been straight-jacketed to the rest of the foot inside shoes. When we walk around, we are constantly and subtly jamming our feet forward into that closed diamond shape that defines most footwear, squeezing our toes together into an unnatural pattern. And as we spend our lives walking on flat surfaces, we rarely evert our feet in response to changes in terrain. So the peroneus longus doesn't do much. In lots of people, it may kind of be asleep. And if it's asleep, it can't do an effective job stabilizing the outside of the knee. The failure to activate the muscles through motion in the foot can, in this way, lead to their failure to perform their other functions as well.

This phenomenon is not exclusive to the peroneus longus. There's a lot going on down there around your ankles, but it can be illustrative to investigate this particular muscle and its function within the pose.

Stabilizing the ankles in Vitruvian Person forces the peroneus longus muscles to contract and bring the ankle joint back to neutral. For many people, this will take time and focus. That's fine. We simply explore the way your patterns respond to the pose and then repattern accordingly.

---

[93] Lift the outer edge of the foot upward toward the outer shin.

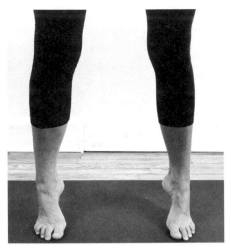 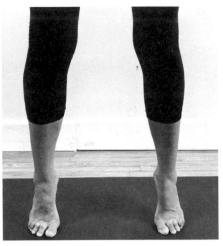

Here the feet are rolled outward, putting the weight of the pose into the outer ankles.   *Line up the feet and ankles by drilling the balls of the feet downward into the mat.*

BREATHING

Notice how the bottom of a full exhalation roots to the bottom of your spine, how the muscles around your pelvis activate. Use that engagement to establish stability in the position.

OPTIONS

If you're feeling stable, lift your arms overhead and reach for the ceiling. (No back bending, please.) If you're feeling both stable and fancy, once your arms are up, do spirit fingers. (Keep in mind, those are not spirit fingers. *These* are spirit fingers.[94])

GOALS

* develop stability in the hips and ankles
* develop leg and glutes strength
* develop mindful balance

---

[94] If you don't get it, I'm sorry. If you get it, I'm sorry.

Mid-Stance Fold

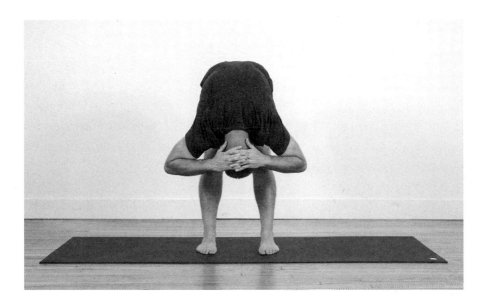

SETUP

Come down from Vitruvian Person and put your hands on your hips. Line up your feet so they're pointing forward. (Feet turned out a little bit is fine here too. Feel it out.)

Bend your knees a bit.

ENTRANCE

Inhale: Take your elbows back, lift your heart, and look up.
Between: Bend your knees deeply.
Exhale: Heart-first, bring your upper body down and fold yourself between your legs.

Let your hands drop to the floor for a moment. Hang down "like a drunk on a fence".[95]

---

[95] This is an actual quote from Richard Freeman, a master Ashtanga teacher. Perhaps the most effective metaphor I've ever heard in a yoga class.

After a breath, interlace your hands behind your head. Make sure they're on the back of your skull, not your neck. Don't pull or anything; that would be weird. Just let yourself be.

ASSESSMENT

If you're drifting back into your heels, reestablish the balls of your feet into the mat. And while we're at it, notice how the weight of your body is landing in your feet. Notice if you're rolling the weight to the inner or outer edges, and work to distribute things a bit more evenly. Remember the tripod of the foot: ball, pinkie toe mound, heel.

Keep a gentle bend in the knees.

More often than not people tend to stare at the floor in this one, activating the posterior chain and gripping the back of the neck. See if you can let the neck soften and release the weight of the skull down toward the floor. Allow for a sense of softness in the upper palate, at the roof of your mouth.

Grip the back of your neck softly. Don't try to yank your own head off (we'll get to that later); just let the weight of your hands coax the skin of your skull softly toward the ground. (What a Cronenberg body-horror sentence that was. I'm so sorry.)

THE ATLANTO-OCCIPITAL JOINT AND THE HUMAN STRESS RESPONSE

You ever go to scary movies? You know the part called the "jump scare"? Where something hops out of the darkness at inhuman speed and comes at the screen with eyes wide and white and your fingers go jangly as you scream and maybe pee a little? When you do that, what happens in your neck? It gets all bound up in the back, right?

You scrunch the back of your neck when you're freaked out to protect the back of your neck from something like a tiger or a basilisk. Since your eyes and hands are oriented forward, the fastest way to defend the back of your neck—the most vulnerable spot on the back of your body—is a high-speed shrug. Your neck tenses in a kind of "protect the vitals" motion, which is part of your stress response.

What happens when your source of stress is not a tiger that you can escape, but something ongoing and oppressive, like the President of the United States on Twitter? Well, in some ways your body responds similarly. It still activates that physical "protect the vitals" action, just more subtly and for a longer time.

One of the most visible places this shows up is the atlanto-occipital joint, or AO joint, in the back of the neck, where the top of your neck (the atlas bone) meets the back of the skull (the occipital bone). This is the space where support and movement of the spine interacts with the stable, heavy weight that is the head. It is a highly dynamic and important joint, allowing for a wide range of motion while also protecting your brain stem. When we have great emotional stress, muscular tension can "grip" around the AO joint, which can sometimes cause issues like tension headaches.

Remember that a major function of the spine is to support the head, so you might consider the AO joint as a sort of keystone or microcosm of this whole structure. If you focus on this spot, you may start to discover that small changes in tension and sensation there are reverberative; information communicates both to and from this point throughout the spine. You may also find that a great deal of unconscious tension is hiding there. Some of this may be emotional stress; some of it may be the result of forward head carriage, or maybe both.

Develop a habit of checking into that spot, taking a look at it, and seeing what happens when you mindfully allow it to relax. When we say things like "neck, jaw, teeth, tongue, roof of the mouth, base of the skull," we are, in part, targeting this area with attention in an attempt to release unnecessary tension. I have had many students who have discovered a major transition in their practices by regularly sending their awareness toward the AO joint.

BREATHING

This is a good opportunity, following the engaged decompression breathing in Vitruvian Person, to let the breathing completely relax. Feel the wave of breath moving in your back body especially. Think of your head like a bowling ball at the end of a bungee cord. Let it be heavy so the spine can gently lengthen into gravity.

OPTIONS

There are several good options for the position of your arms in this position. Play around with them and make the posture suit your own needs.

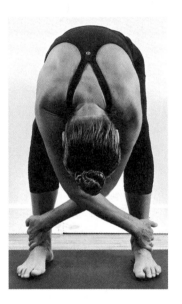

1. Cross-armed: With your right hand, take your left ankle. With your left hand, take your right ankle. Steadily bend both arms as you let your head hang loose.

2. Spider-Man: On tented fingers, walk your hands back between your legs as far as you can. Gently tuck your chin to complete the rounding of your whole spine. (Remember to keep a little bend in the knees.)

GOALS

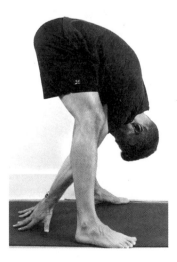

* relaxed spinal decompression
* relaxed hip opening
* gentle lengthening of the posterior chain
* release of the AO joint

Warrior 2

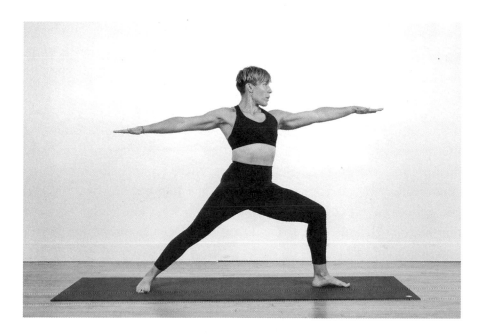

SETUP

Take a wide-legged stance and turn your right foot out 90 degrees, just like you would if you were going to do Warrior 2. Bring your arms out wide.

Set your back foot at about a 45-degree angle. *About*—don't be overly geometric about this; we want to find a steady position for your foot with your heel down comfortably.

ENTRANCE

Inhale: Let your arms float a bit and open your chest.
Exhale: Gently bend your right knee to the lunge.

ASSESSMENT

Take your back (left) arm and swing it forward so it is in line with your right hand. Line up your arms with your lunging leg so your hands, arms, right femur, right foot, and your eyes are all pointing the same direction.

Now make both of your hands into fists and squeeze tight. Imagine you've got a heavy-duty trash bag (unused, fresh out of the box, it's cool) in your hands. Pull your left hand back across your chest and tear the trash bag apart. Don't just mime it either. Engage the resistance of this sixteen-ply Glad bag. Put some muscle into it. With your right hand pushing forward and your left drawing back, try to find an engaged connection between your hands, across the line of your heart. When you release the hands from their gripped position and make them the familiar blade-shape of Warrior 2, see if you can maintain the length and tension of this line.

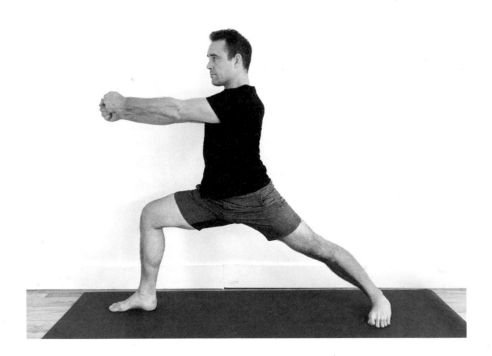

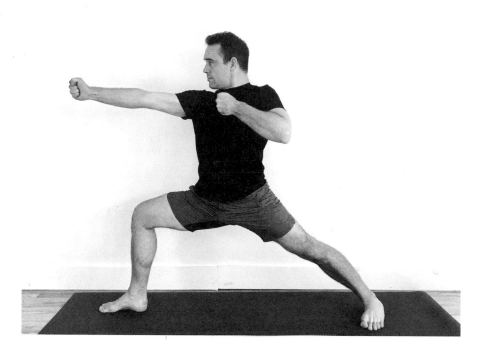

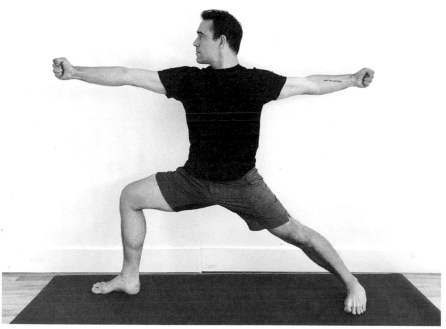

More than anything, mindfully maintain the line of your lunging knee. The pose is built upon this structure and as things progress—especially to the Warrior Triangle (next)—the knee may try to dip inward. Keep it steady and build outward from there.

Notice if your core is releasing and starting to sink in a back bend. "Zip up" the belly, drawing your navel back and up to stabilize the lower spine. Notice again the connection between front body stability and back body compression. If you've got effective abdominal support, you'll have better luck getting your lower spine to decompress.

On your right foot, notice your toes. If they're grabbing the floor, ungrip a bit. You don't need to hold the ground beneath you; you won't float away. Instead, firmly ground your right heel, like you could put your energy down beneath the floor. You may notice that when you do this, the right hip begins to engage more strongly.

With your back leg, do the straw-smoothie thing. Imagine trying to pull the floor up through your left leg like peanut butter through a straw. Feel how this engages the strength of your leg all the way to the pelvic floor.

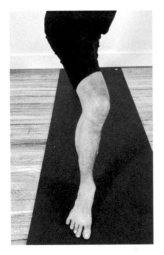

It is quite common for students to twist the knee inward when setting into the lunge.

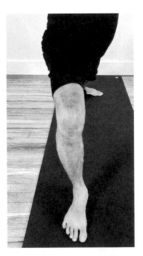

Align the knee with the foot to the best of your ability, so it is not twisted inward. This may require that you adjust your hips forward.

Oh, yeah. Also: easy with your face there, killer. This is a peaceful warrior. Relax your jaw and let your head float. Notice the roof of your mouth and see if you can allow for a sense of softness there. Once you're set nicely, reengage the central structure of the pose: the legs and hips.

BREATHING

Move the inhales into your back and use the exhales to firmly stabilize your core, especially at the very bottom of your spine. In time, the inhale can rise through the entire rib cage—front and back—and the exhale can work to maintain the "lift" of the upper body.

OPTIONS

This one is pretty straightforward. However, if you are working to maintain Healthy Neutral in the pelvis and have healthy knees, experiment with gently bending your back leg a bit. This position can make your knee a bit vulnerable, so go gently. You may find it helps you to stabilize your pelvis and engage the muscles of your right thigh more fully.

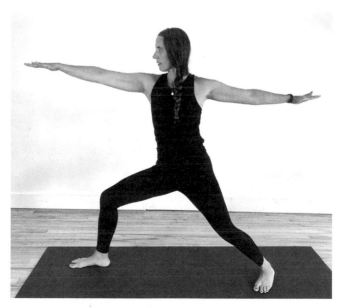

Bending the back knee in Warrior 2 allows the pelvis more movement and can allow greater access to Healthy Neutral.

GOALS

- strengthen the right (lunging) leg and hip
- pattern hip stability and mobility in an open lunge
- pattern Healthy Neutral and spinal decompression in the core
- open the shoulders and chest

Warrior Triangle

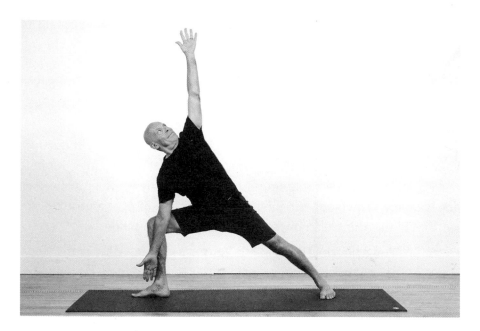

SETUP

From Warrior 2, turn your palms forward, thumbs up. With both hands, put the tips of your fingers against the shoulders of imaginary soccer players. Push them apart. Stretch the line across your heart as widely as it goes.

Stay strongly anchored in your right heel.

ENTRANCE

Lean your torso over your right thigh and move your arms so that your right wrist lines up with the inside of your right knee. Start there; don't go too low.

Our primary line for this pose is not measured by your arm and knee, it is measured by your torso and rear leg. Establish a clean line from your left ankle to your left shoulder, best you can.

Keeping the back of your neck long, gently sweep your chin toward your left shoulder. Notice if your neck—or face—starts to grip here. If you can't turn your head all the way to 90 degrees, just do what you can. (The tendency here is to cheat the neck into hyperextension to get the chin all the way to the shoulder, so your head is kind of falling off behind you. Maintain a neutral position in the neck and go to a comfortable depth.)

ASSESSMENT

Check the line of your lunge. As the weight of the upper body shifts over your lunging leg, there will be a temptation to cheat by sticking your butt out behind you and sinking into a localized backbend. Keep your core engaged and remember, the lunge is the foundation of the posture. We can't build this thing effectively if we're not well-grounded.

+ Speaking of which, check out your toes again. Ungrip the floor. Stay strongly rooted in your right heel.

+ Just as in Warrior 2, "zip up" the belly with special focus on the lower abdomen. Notice if you're driving the ribs out to hang in the back bend.

BREATHING

Heart-opening inhales, without back-bending. Steady core-engaging exhales, without gripping your neck.

OPTIONS

+ Only take the lunge as deeply as you can, maintaining your healthy line, back leg through spine. If that means you only bend the knee a bit, that's fine. You can increase the depth of the pose by deepening the lunge then reestablishing the line of your torso.

+ If you can establish Healthy Neutral through the spine, you might explore the intermediate form by taking the lunge all the way down to a half squat. Keep your right arm inside your leg and bend your knee as deeply as you comfortably can. Reach your right palm as close to the floor as you can, far away, without touching it. Hover your palm above the floor like you're feeling for the heat of a dying campfire. Now, lift the outer edge of your back foot so its sole comes away from the floor. This half squat is challenging; don't push too far. The exit is particularly tough: press your right heel firmly and bring yourself up until your right leg is straight.

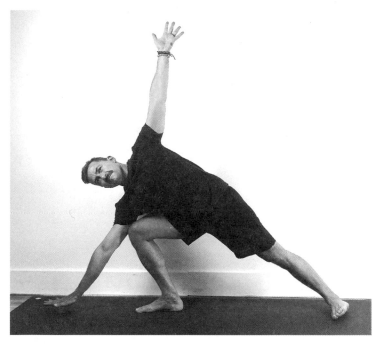

Notice Chris's back foot here. See how he's lifting the outer edge so the bottom of his foot is peeled away from the floor? That's the good stuff, right there.

GOALS

- strengthen the lunging leg and hip
- integrate the myofascia of the left (rear) leg with that of the left side of the torso
- pattern hip stability in a broad, challenging position
- open the chest
- pattern neutral breathing in diagonal lean

Pyramid

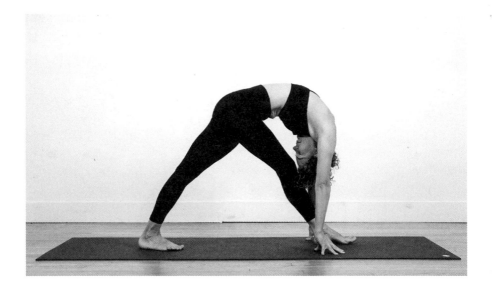

SETUP

From a neutral standing position, step your left leg back in a short lunge.

Plant the left heel down to the ground so your back foot is turned 30–45 degrees outward. Set your feet in their own lanes, so they're not crossed up. Now square your hips forward toward your right foot.

ENTRANCE

This one has a few phases, synced with breath.

Inhale: Lift your arms overhead.
Exhale: Bring your arms forward and knit your ribs.

Now make strong fists with both hands like you're grabbing a rowing machine.

Inhale: Draw the handles of the rowing machine back, all the way to the sides of the rib cage.

Exhale: Bring your upper body down halfway so you're relatively level with the floor.

Inhale: Hold here.

Exhale: Put your hands to the floor, just forward of your right foot.

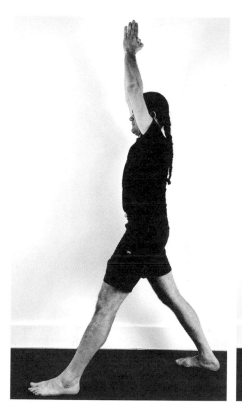
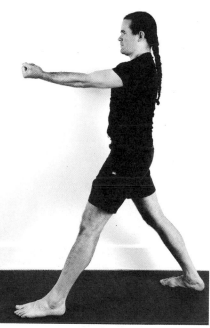

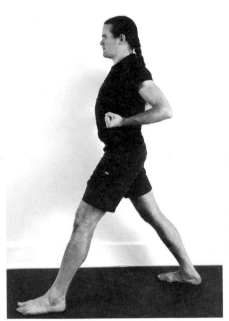

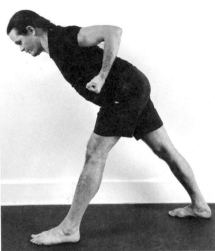

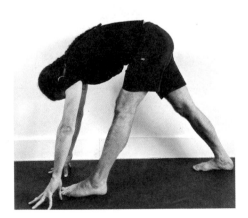

Pause a moment to clear your neck.

Inhale: Bend both knees deeply and look forward.
Exhale: Tuck your tailbone to round your spine as you straighten your right leg.

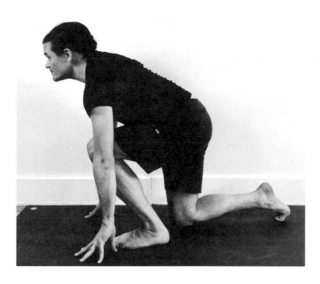

To complete the entrance, tuck your chin and move your forehead toward your right knee. Press your fingertips into the ground and lift your navel.

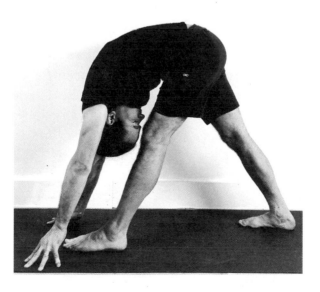

ASSESSMENT

Ground the ball of the right foot strongly and keep the toes ungripped.

Notice the right side of the torso. It tends to shorten a good deal as we enter this. Think about the posture "hips-out," meaning we try to establish a healthy position in the hips first, then work outward from there.[96] Likewise, we can think about progress in the position hips-first; focus on the tuck of your tailbone inside the position and you may discover ripple effects in your core strength and access to spinal flexion.

BREATHING

Oh, boy. This one. The idea for the breathing here isn't complicated, but making it happen takes a good amount of focus. We want to first acknowledge, then increase, the compression of the front body in this position. In many ways this means freeing up space in the posterior chain for you to breathe. And for those of us who are still working on finding space and movement in the posterior chain—and frankly the rest of us too—this can be a challenge.

So maybe do less. Not less breathing; less depth. Take yourself to something like 85 percent of your capacity and explore moving breath inside compact positions. There's an opportunity here to explore a certain perspective on yoga poses, in which the body is like the bed of a river or the curve of a half pipe on Venice Beach; it is a boundary for motion and action within. I'll refrain from getting esoteric or metaphysical here and simply invite you into the idea that a yoga pose is a boundary for the motion of your breath. This motion follows the curvature of your physical being, it carves the hollows and rides the edges across interior space. And just like water in a riverbed, in time the breath can establish depth and wash away obstacles to find a smoother, more direct line of flow.

This is an idea. Try it on. When you enter a yoga pose, you might think, *This is how I embrace the breath.* See what happens.

---

[96] Part of this is because we aren't working with Healthy Neutral in the spine nearly as much in this pose. Obviously the spine is in deep flexion, so we build our assessment of the pose from a more localized part of the body.

HEAD-FIRST YOGA

The neck, for healthy human beings, is the most mobile portion of the spine. When we walk around the world, we are constantly adjusting the position of the head to maintain balance and observe the world around us. So it's only natural for us to originate much of our intentional movement from our head. When you walk around a corner, usually your head will turn a bit before your chest and hips, as you check with your eyes to see where your body is going.

This tendency can find its way into your yoga practice. In front-side compressions like Pyramid, it's fairly common for students to use a tuck in the chin as the central, driving action. You may find greater success if you reverse this tendency and think about originating the action from your hips instead. Starting the "tuck" from your tailbone encourages the abdominal muscles to engage more fully and more directly targets the lower back for opening.

This is an investigation, not an edict. Just check it out. When moving into spinal flexion (or any position, really), experiment with moving hips-first instead of skull-first. Notice what parts of the body activate. You might find greater access to and benefits from many of your poses.

OPTIONS

We often do a version of this one that's pretty much the first stage of a pose called Flamingo. We call it "The Weird One."[97] In this variation, first walk your hands back behind your right foot. Spin them around and go up on tented fingertips. Next, lift your back heel so you're up on your toes. Then bend your back leg and bring both knees in line. (They might not actually get in line, just aim in that direction.)

---

[97] Tried to make "weird-amid," the combo of *weird* and *pyramid*, work for a while. No dice. It's too dumb to take seriously and not dumb enough to really stick. (For an example of "so dumb it stuck," see: the Stamos.

You'll find this orientation takes a lot more core engagement, which is good.

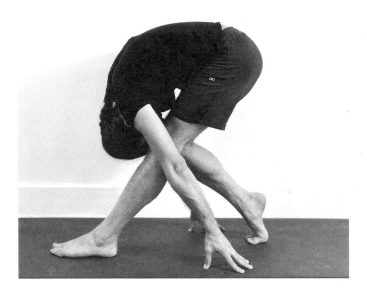

If you can do the Weird One with a good degree of stability, you can take this even further to Flamingo Pose. Try lifting your back heel up to your butt. Make sure you don't shift your hips forward too far, which makes it more of a forward fold. Instead, use your hands and front leg to create a sort of tripod for support. Then breathe.

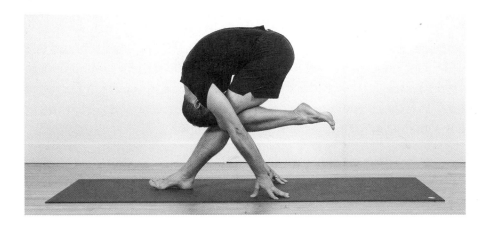

GOALS

- compress the front side body and strengthen abdominal muscles
- open the muscles of the back
- open the right hamstrings
- open the right hip
- open the left ankle
- develop stability and control throughout the spine, particularly around the pelvis

Revolved Triangle

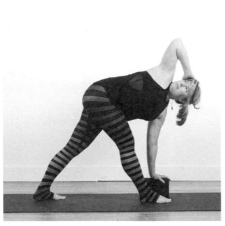
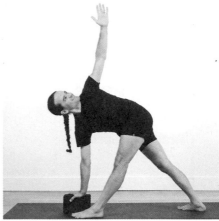

SETUP

From Pyramid, lift your head up to come out of the rounded position. Set your left hand on the floor (or a block) and make the connection there strong and stable. Get your torso level (ish) to the floor.

Place your right hand in Stamos, palm to the back of your skull. (If Stamos doesn't work for you, your hand on your sacrum is also good.)

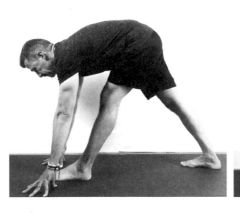
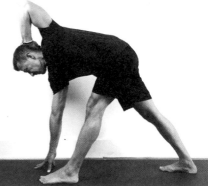

ENTRANCE

Inhale: Draw your spine long.

Exhale: Lift your right elbow up and open your chest to the right.

ASSESSMENT

Keep the ball of your right (front) foot grounded, toes ungripped.

If your right hip is swinging forward—so your right-side body is shortened—gently draw it back to move toward an even position in the torso, right to left.

As, you know, pretty much always, notice if you're gripping the back of your neck. Especially if you're trying to look up to the ceiling here, there's a tendency to grip the neck into hyperextension. Maintain neutral and turn your head to the degree it's available; that's all.

Keep your right hand in Stamos. (We used to teach this one with the arm reaching up to start, but in time we had to let that go. The desire and attempt to reach to the ceiling got in the way, because it provides a compelling illusion that the pose has really developed and opened. But more often than not this is just that: an illusion.) Stamos is a no-nonsense position. It doesn't allow much cheating. For this reason, you might (probably?) hate it. That's cool. Foundations isn't here to win popularity contests; it's here to raise money for Derek's pancreatic surgery with the most epic bake sale the Chattanooga High Devil-Bats have ever seen.

Wait. That's not it either. (Although it would be a wonderful goal; Derek is a great guy.)

What I mean is, depth isn't the point. Instagram is not the point. "Getting there" isn't the point. If something works, maybe we don't need to push it. Maybe it just works and we can leave it at that.

BREATHING

Just let it move in this one. The twist is a very effective container for the breath. You can potentially explore an "inhale-lengthen, exhale-twist" action, if you like. You can choose. Just know that simply breathing is enough. (This is also a decent notion for life in general.)

OPTIONS

- If you have freakish gorilla arms like me, you might be comfortable doing this one without a block.
- To do the intermediate form, float your left hand off the floor and make both hands into fists. Press them away, punching outward into the air.
- I'm not even going to tell you what the advanced form of this pose is because then you'll try it.

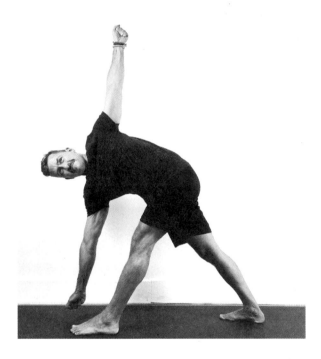

GOALS

- pattern healthy rotation through the torso
- open the front leg's hamstring
- open the back leg's ankle
- stabilize the upper back (particularly on the right)
- pattern stability in the hips

Tree Pose

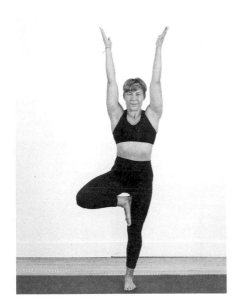 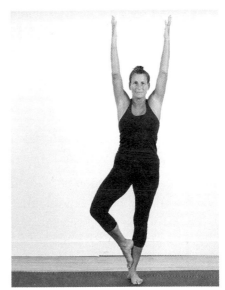

SETUP

From standing, put a little bounce in your knees. Shift to your left foot with the weight trending toward your heel.

Place your hands on your hips, thumbs over your glutes, and lift your chest up.

ENTRANCE

Set your right foot on the inside of your left calf.

Bring your hands together at your heart center with the thumbs resting gently against your sternum.

Stand tall.

ASSESSMENT

◆ Like in the other balancing postures, especially Big Toe Pose, Tree is meant, for us at least, to train the body to stand upright. After the opening provided by the other standing poses, you may find healthy posture a bit more available to you. Take advantage of this opportunity to pattern neutral into the system: ribs in, heart high, neck ramped, jaw soft, weight trending over the heel.

- Find something like a plumb line, the best you can. Think *knee over ankle, hip over knee, heart over hips, head over heart.* You might discover that doing this pose, while holding Healthy Neutral in the spine, is no small challenge. Most people have a bit of repatterning to do to reestablish Healthy Neutral human posture. And that's cool. That's what we're here for.

- Notice the hips might want to push forward, so they're over the toes. See if you can keep yourself in the plumb line.

- It's very common to swing the right knee out to the side as wide as you can. Resist this impulse. Notice that if you swing your knee too far to the side, your hips will start to spin in that direction as well. Imagine you have headlights on your hips and keep them pointed straight down the road in front of you. Only move the knee out as far as is available without swinging the headlights to the right.

- Think for a moment of a water fountain that shoots water straight up in a vertical line. (Sort of like those bird baths, you know?) And imagine a little orange ping-pong ball balanced right on the top of that lovely vertical stream. That orange ball? That's your head. Let it rest, nicely supported by the upward flow of energy through your spine.

- The common metaphor for Tree Pose is to imagine you're a … tree. And you root down beneath the earth in all directions and slowly rise toward the sun from that support. I really want to hate this metaphor (recall: I am a hipster) but I can't. It's about as effective as they come. So, yeah, imagine you're a tree.

BREATHING

- Since the posture is upright, you can play around with things without much resistance. I love exploring the area of the kidney wings here, since it's a less intuitive place to breathe than, say, the space of collarbones.

- If you're having issues keeping the ribs in, use your exhales to stabilize the core muscles.

OPTIONS

◆ If you can maintain Healthy Neutral in your spine, especially at your ribs, then you might explore taking your arms overhead. You can put hands in prayer, take them shoulder width apart, or "hold the sphere." Whichever you like; just make sure that chasing the upward lift in the hands and arms isn't getting in the way of Healthy Neutral.

◆ I sometimes like to tell people to wave their arms like kelp in the tide. The idea here is, if you can hold your hips stable in any given standing position, you can move your upper body around without losing balance. If the upper body has a solid foundation, then it can just play. (We know this from just day-to-day life. You can stand on two feet and wave your arms around, no problem. If you stand on one foot and wave your arms, it gets harder. The difference is that, essentially, two grounded legs stabilize your hips much better than one. But if you learn to stabilize the pelvis while on one leg—which takes a lot of hip strength, unless you're sitting in your joints—you can do all kinds of weird stuff with your arms and head.)

◆ Extra challenge: If you're all like, "Tree Pose is lame and basic. Can we do arm balances or whatever, please? I'm bored." Then, OK … first off, watch the attitude. This is a yoga book. Second, try this. Once you're set in the pose, close your eyes. Count fifteen slow breaths.[98]

GOALS

◆ pattern Healthy Neutral in a moderately challenged position
◆ strengthen the standing leg
◆ balance, balance, balance

---

[98] If you did this and it wasn't hard, then, OK, gauntlet thrown. Well played. Now go up on your toes and close your eyes.

Corpse (a.k.a. Savasana)

Lie down on your back with your palms up and your heart open. Let your legs be relaxed. Close your eyes and breathe the air. Five to ten easy breaths, here.[99]

---

[99] This particular Savasana is affectionately known in our community as the "Betsy Baker Savasana." Betsy is a Foundations teacher who, in the early days, advocated for additional moments of rest in the sequence. That was a smart move. So we named it after her. This tradition is the reason we're referencing the Sanskrit name for the pose here.

FEELING FOR THINGS

Imagine for a moment that you're taking a walk in the park with a good friend. And you're talking about, I don't know, the sudden reemergence of Devon Sawa on the cultural radar sometime around the music video for Eminem's classic song "Stan" and those Final Destination movies, after which he promptly returned to obscurity. Got it? OK. Cool.

So, you're talking about Mr. Sawa, and you're pretty wrapped up in it, because you were a fan. (Weren't we all?) But then, just as you're holding forth about how sometimes a performer's passion can elevate otherwise trivial material, your friend stops you and says, "Hey! Look at the birds!" And you do stop. And you do look at the birds. There they are, flying overhead. Maybe it's a murmuration of starlings, in which case you're now probably having a quasi-religious experience. Regardless, you stop and you look at the birds.

Here's what I'm not going to say. I'm not going to say, *Thank God for your friend who obviously knows how to be "present" and reminded you to do the same.* We aren't here to make that kind of value judgment.

What I will say is this: the human mind is, by its nature, very bad at holding two thoughts at once. (None of us are actually that good at multitasking, it turns out.) Noticing the birds and making a point about Mr. Sawa's transition from child star to Hollywood upstart—these things can't really be done at the same time. Not very well, at least. Your friend simply interrupted one stream of attention and put you into another, so you could see and experience something you might have otherwise missed.

This is, in many ways, what good yoga teachers do. They reorient the way that you're seeing things. I don't necessarily mean they reformat the rotation of your chakras, I just mean they point things out. They invite you to step off one train of attention and onto another, because it's not really possible for your mind to fully focus on lunch plans and hamstring pain at the same time.

Here's something that's happened to all of us, I'm sure: you're working really hard in a pose, something that you've been holding for a while or you're attempting for the first time, and your teacher walks up to you as if to offer detailed, refined guidance, and she just says, "Hey. Breathe." And suddenly you realize you were holding your breath the whole time. That's weird, right? How do we miss that?

Leaving aside the biomechanics, or the parts about anxiety and stress response while under physical strain, when you stop to think about it, it's pretty wild that at some point in the practice many of us will simply *stop breathing without even noticing it*. But it happens all the time. This significant event—and it is a significant event, holding your breath—happens without your permission and goes on without you noticing. Attention is funny this way. Good yoga teachers, as far as I can tell, are the ones who understand their students' needs and have the ability to identify what they may be missing within their present attention.

When I say, "Feel your neck and your lower back," I invite you to really dig in. Get off whatever train of attention you're on, especially if it's the "go as high as I can" train, and explore the sensations inside your back bend. This is a primary benefit of the practice. It trains the mind to "feel" shapes effectively and respond in kind.

In time, the work of repatterning allows many of the details of practice to become second nature. You will need less and less attention to stand upright in healthy posture, because your body will have the pattern for it drilled deep into the soft tissue. At that point, you'll be able to stop focusing on physical posture and get back to pointless nostalgic pop-culture analysis.

Supine Sequence

Wind Removing

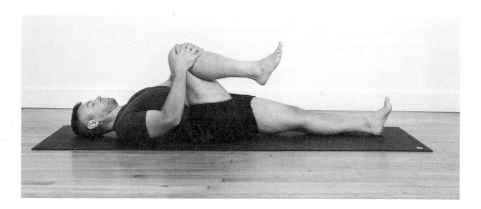

SETUP

From Corpse Pose, bring your right knee up to your chest and grab hold of it with both hands.

ENTRANCE

Inhale: Broaden your shoulders.
Exhale: Steadily pull your right knee toward your right shoulder.

ASSESSMENT

Use the ground here to measure Healthy Neutral. What you'll likely find is your shoulders try to round forward. If that's happening, take a moment to imagine your shoulders in this position while standing up, and notice you're in a textbook shoulder hunch. Draw your shoulders wide, opening the line of your heart. At the same time, lengthen the back of your neck as if to flatten it on the floor, and look down your nose toward your heart.

While there is a good degree of general hip opening in this pose, we might consider the upper body as its primary focus. Establishing the position of your right leg is fairly straightforward, but getting your upper back to engage and your neck to flatten requires—for many of us—consistent, mindful attention.

You might explore engaged resistance here. Push your right knee into your grip, like you're trying to move it away from your chest, while pulling against the knee strongly with your hands. You can choose how much resistance you give yourself here. Just make sure you're not pushing yourself into struggle, or you lose the work in your neck and shoulders.

BREATHING

Send the breath to your right hip, to explore the ways we can move tissue and energy around there.

OPTIONS

If you feel any pinching in your right hip, modify the position of your right leg.[100] If you're on the flexible side of the spectrum, try guiding your knee outward on a diagonal line from the center. (A good way to think of this is: instead of taking your knee to your right shoulder, take it to your right bicep.) If you're feeling closely, you may begin to find a natural outward curve at the front of your pelvis. Follow this curve, letting your thigh and knee track outward from the midline of your body.

In terms of functional movement, this outward movement of the thigh when the hip is in deep flexion makes perfect sense—it doesn't do much good for you to knee yourself in the chest while scaling a boulder or climbing a tree. If you're going to use such a large range of motion, it follows that at a certain point your leg would begin to swing wide of the

------

[100] For many years I taught and practiced "find the pinch; the pinch is good." But it turns out the pinch isn't good. The pinch is your body telling you you're putting too much pressure on the iliac crest, which can wear down some important connective tissue that guards the hip. And that is bad.

torso to avoid smacking you in the rib cage. (Stop hitting yourself, quoth the sages. Stop hitting yourself.)

Two variations for the grip that may be helpful to explore:

1. One-handed: If you're flexible in the hip and your knee is starting to track outward, you might release the left hand from the grip. Place it on your left hip, and use it to help keep your pelvis relatively level against the floor. Let your right hand maintain a grip at the right knee to guide it into the pose.

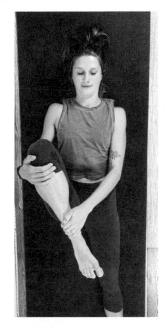

2. Knee and ankle: Keeping your right hand on your knee, place your left hand on your right ankle. Let your right shin gently move to a diagonal, knee away from the midline. Keep the toes of your right foot active, especially the pinky toe, to help stabilize your knee. Then add resistance: with your hands, pull your shin in and up toward your heart; with your shin, push away. Notice how this engages your right hip, as your external rotators—primarily your glutes—have to kick in to do the "push away" action at your knee and shin.

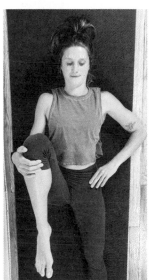

GOALS

- ◆ open the hips
- ◆ strengthen the upper back and the front of the neck
- ◆ open the hip flexors
- ◆ maybe strengthen the biceps, if you're using your resistance

Wind Removing (Both Legs)

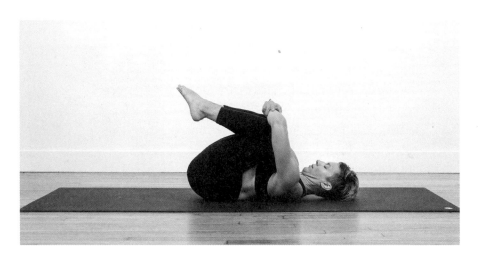

SETUP

From Savasana, draw both legs up to your chest. Wrap yourself up in a ball, hands clasped over knees.

ENTRANCE

Take a deep breath. As you exhale, tuck your chin and try to lift your forehead to touch your knees. It's fine if you can't get there. Just do what's available to you. As compact as possible.

Take another deep breath in this position, feeling your back body expand. As you exhale, slowly roll your spine down to the floor.

ASSESSMENT

There's a temptation to pull on your knees in this one. Don't: more likely than not you'll begin to grip around the systems we are trying to open, like your lower back and neck. Instead, simply establish the grip strongly with your hands and give the pose a gentle hug. Then just breathe. This position will drive the breath into the back body by itself, so don't add too much effort.

Look down your nose toward your heart, feeling the back of your neck lengthen down toward the floor. You don't have to make contact with the back of your neck; we're just going for the basic motion.

Feel and allow for the compression of your abdomen.

Keep the jaw soft.

INVESTIGATIVE BREATHING

One of the processes we encourage in Foundations is called Investigative Breathing. Investigative Breathing is the opposite of what we might call "prescriptive" breathing, where we try to modify tension patterns through breathing practice. We have looked at a lot of Prescriptive Breathing techniques so far; now let's check out the alternative style. In Investigative Breathing we use the breath as a vehicle for discovery. It's the difference between an explorer and a farmer: one maps the territory, the other cultivates it to suit a specific goal.

When you take a full breath, it moves and manipulates your body in ways that are unique to you. The motion of the breath follows your personal tension patterns, like water follows ravines and gullies downhill. With every breath you have an opportunity to explore your own internal shapes: the lines of flow and the lines of obstruction, where things narrow down and where they open up. When we simply let the breath do what it "wants," we are allowed to observe its path of least resistance. While it's not always the single best approach, Investigative Breathing can be illuminative. It brings light to the internal darkness, the parts of ourselves that we can't usually see.

Following the Rule of Three, we understand the value of both Investigative and Prescriptive Breathing. They are two approaches to the practice, each with their own value. When one isn't providing insight or progress for you in a particular part of your practice, try the other. Play with both and see what comes up.

BREATHING

Just let it move.

OPTIONS

If wrapping up is difficult, throw a strap across your knees and hold that. It's fine to just put your hands on your knees, but that's not quite as effective. If you can close the chain between your arms, it will allow you to relax your shoulders down a bit more.

GOALS

- ◆ open the hips and the muscles of the back
- ◆ decompress the spine in a passive position, primarily through breathing

Bridge

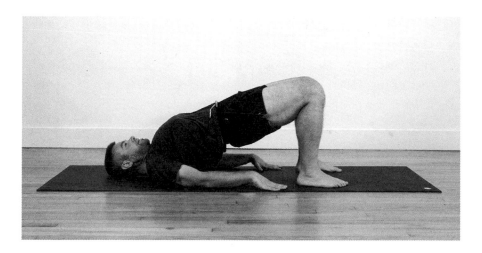

SETUP

From Wind Removing, place your feet flat on the ground. Keep them generally hip-width and generally parallel, but no need to be exact. (Remember your body is uniquely constructed, so geometrical standards might not truly meet your personal needs.)

Put your arms by your sides, palms down on the mat and shoulders broad. Let your head rest on the floor.

If you've got a yoga block, put it between your knees.

ENTRANCE

Inhale: Press your hands and arms down into the mat.
Exhale: Knit your ribs down and push the mid-back into the mat.
Notice this will begin to tuck your tailbone upward and engage your abdominal muscles.
Inhale: Open the breath into the chest while keeping your tailbone tucked.
Exhale: Follow this tuck of the tailbone and lift one vertebra at a time off the floor, until you're up on your shoulders with your back off the mat.

ASSESSMENT

Keep your chin a bit away from your chest. If you start to feel a stretching sensation in your neck, ease up. As a general rule, we don't want to stretch your neck while it's under significant load.[101]

When you're getting into your Bridge, we take a hips-first approach. The tuck of the tailbone will help us keep the back bend from becoming overly localized around the mid-back.[102] It'll take a lot of power in your glutes to keep from dropping into the back bend once you're lifted in the position, so get ready for a ride.

In time we can work on the heart-opening portion of this pose, but only once we have firmly established Healthy Neutral around the pelvis and mid-back.

If you have a block, squeeze it with your knees. Remember, your adductors help stabilize your pelvis, so if you keep them active, it will help you maintain Healthy Neutral around the hips.

If you don't have a block, just keep your knees about hip width.

Ungrip your toes from the floor.

BREATHING

The placement of the breath largely depends on how well we can maintain relative neutral in the hips. If you're finding the back bend is getting localized, focus on inhaling into your back and tucking the tailbone with the exhale.

If you can hold the hips toward relative neutral and you're not in a localized back bend, start using your inhales to open your chest. As soon as you start doing this, you may notice the back bend starts to localize. So, you may have to go back and forth between stabilizing the hips and opening the chest. The inhale-exhale cycle works well for this. Inhale to open the chest, exhale to tuck the tailbone.

---

[101] Neck injuries in poses like Shoulder Stand and Plow are not uncommon, often because students place the load of the body directly onto the back of the neck. Your neck is not really designed to carry that kind of load by itself.

[102] The thoracolumbar junction, the most mobile portion of the spine outside of your neck.

DEEP FRONT LINE BREATHING

In his book *Anatomy Trains,* Thomas Myers identifies the deep front line (DFL), an integrated myofascial train that runs from the feet to the skull "deep" in the body. This line includes the adductors, hip flexors, QLs, the respiratory diaphragm, the pulmonary pleurae, the longus colli, the longus capitis, and the scalenes.[103]

The deep front line is the primary vessel for the "wave" of breath through the body. Unfortunately, if we look at the structures that lose integration and power from sedentary life, we will find most of the DFL on the list. Reactivating the DFL in a well-integrated manner can be a powerful method for restoring balance in breath and movement.

In Bridge we can do good work toward reactivating the DFL with what we call deep front line breathing. All you do is reach your arms straight up toward the sky, far as you can. Imagine you're really trying to give a beach ball to God. Now knit your low ribs in, tuck your tail, squeeze the block with your knees, and breathe as deeply as is available.

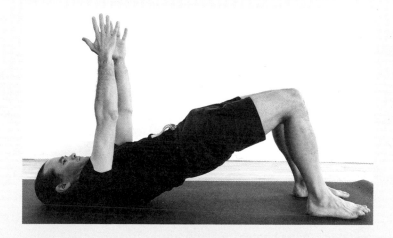

---

[103] Vitally, these last three muscle groups are responsible for correcting hyperextension in the neck. If you've got forward head carriage, you'll want to do some work strengthening them.

Here the arm position restricts the top of the rib cage in the breath, but it is difficult to actively breathe in the belly without localizing the back bend. It's a conundrum. In time, you might find that your body starts to resolve this conundrum by moving breath down your back along the line of the QLs.

Hopefully we will begin to feel the mid- and lower back, as well as the adductors, start to engage in the pulse of breath as they are engaged in supporting the body. This is what we're going for: strong activity in the breath while maintaining powerful postural support. Ideally, we will train the DFL to engage fully in the breath while holding you upright at the same time.

Bridge is a good opportunity to explore full exhales. Once you're lifted into the pose, try breathing out as much air as possible. Notice how the hips and lower back may engage strongly at the bottom of the exhale, stabilizing the lower spine. This often requires additional engagement in the hamstrings, which is good. Strong hamstrings are a good goal for your overall practice.

OPTIONS

If you're looking to target the hamstrings and glutes more directly, walk your feet farther away from your hips. The farther you go, the more the hamstrings must support the lift in your hips. This has the added benefit of pulling on the sitz bones,[104] which helps with the tuck of the tail underneath the posture.

Manual adjustments: Once you've set up a well-supported Bridge pose, hook your thumbs around your hips so they're right at the top of your butt. Now use your thumbs to push your glutes toward your knees. Hopefully, you'll feel your hamstrings and glutes fire up as you help coax the pelvis into a tucked neutral position.

---

[104] Ischial tuberosities, my favorite anatomical term.

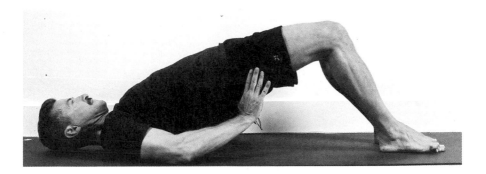

Once you've done that, put your fingertips right at the top of your quads. Slowly push the flesh on your thighs down toward your knees, as if to encourage your quads to contract by pulling *down* instead of *up*.

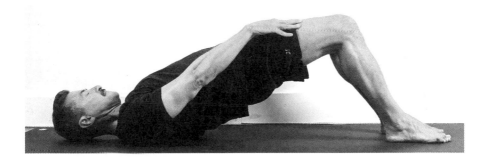

Go back and forth between these two manual adjustments. They can help you establish the strength we are seeking for the posture.

GOALS

- strengthen glutes and thighs, particularly hamstrings
- open the upper chest
- stabilize the core muscles
- strengthen the back
- integrate the deep front line (in DFL breathing)

Plunge

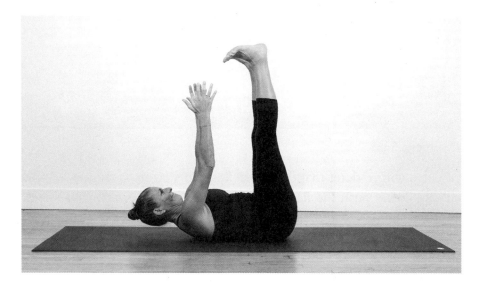

SETUP

Once you're done with Bridge, bring your knees to your shoulders and hold them there with your hands for a moment. Take a breath.

ENTRANCE

Straighten your legs up toward the ceiling. As much as it's available, go for straight and vertical in your legs. If you have short-tight hamstrings, your knees may not straighten all the way. That's fine; just do what's there. If you're bendy, you might find that your legs actually start to lean toward your face. Try to keep them vertical.

Now reach your arms straight up. It should look, from the side, like you're plunging back-first into deep water.

Dorsiflex your ankles as much as you can, driving your heels high in the air. With your hands, reach up like you're trying to give a beach ball to God.

Lock out your elbows and knees here, if you like. (It's safe since the limbs aren't loaded with any real weight, so we're not at a risk of buckling at the elbows or knees.) Feel the tension of the soft tissue wrapping strongly around these joints.

LOCKED SHORT VERSUS LOCKED LONG

When we imagine a muscle being "tight," we often imagine that the tissue is shortened in contraction. You might think of the muscles behind your skull; if the back of your neck is in hyperextension those muscles will "grip" tightly to stabilize your head. And at the same time, they will be in a shortened position. We can call this state "locked short."

This sort of "lock" makes some intuitive sense. If muscles work by contracting, then "loose" muscles would release into a lengthened position. Tight muscles, by definition, are short muscles. Right?

Not really, it turns out. It is possible (and not uncommon) for tight muscles to also be long. When muscle and fascia are lengthened and loaded (i.e., responsible for supporting weight) for a prolonged period of time, they can enter into a state of chronic contraction. When this happens, the muscle tissue will be active—contracting—but not actually *shortening.*

A good example of this is your rhomboids, muscles that hold your shoulder blades stable on your upper back. If you have chronically slouched shoulders,[105] your rhomboids will be in a lengthened position *and* they will be responsible for keeping your shoulder blades from sliding any farther into protraction. In this case it's quite likely that your rhomboids will be both long and tight. The term we use for this is "locked-long."

---

[105] Shoulder blades protracted.

It's important to engage this concept because it's possible for students to feel a muscle is tight and misinterpret the situation. Yes, the muscle is tight—"locked"—but that doesn't always mean the muscle is short. Basically, not all tight muscles need to be stretched. If you have a muscle that is "locked-long," then what it really needs is *strength*[106] more than *stretch*. Being able to tell the difference is important if we are going to address our individual and unique needs in the practice.

---

[106] Or possibly pressure, like in a massage. However, pressure of this sort often involves interventions like massage therapy or myofascial release. Regardless, lengthening the tissue when it is locked-long is usually a bad idea.

ASSESSMENT AND BREATHING

Just feel what it's like to breathe deeply here.

OPTIONS

We can turn this into a core and neck-strengthening position, if you like. It goes like this:

1. Tuck your chin into your neck (mouth closed, please.) Should be giving yourself extra chins right now, hopefully.

2. Pushing your heels to the ceiling, see if you can get your butt to hover off the floor.

3. Keeping your chin tucked, hover your head off the ground. Just hover, like half an inch.

4. Breathe deeply.

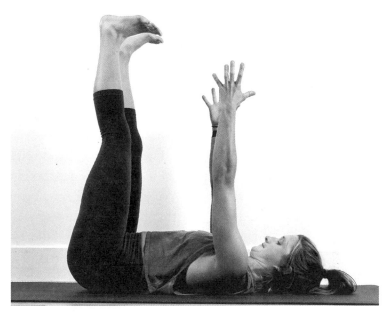

Start in the standard version of Plunge, head and tailbone down.

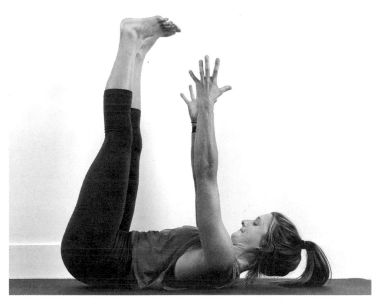

Gently lift the head, keeping the chin tucked, and float the tailbone off the mat.

When practicing this core exercise, you'll likely discover your abdominal wall is working hard and the front of your neck feels fairly intense activation. If you feel your neck getting tight, check into that sensation deeply. I've seen a lot of people get pretty freaked out when they do strength work in their necks, particularly the front-side ones we're working with here. I'm never going to tell you to push through a warning signal from your body. Respect your body. Listen to it. Feed it grapes. If it feels like weird stuff is happening, slow down. However, you might just be discovering a new kind of activation in your neck. Since the neck is a highly sensitive area, you may need to acclimate to this sensation. Take your time, feel it out. Remember that the muscles in the front of your neck are the anti-forward-head-carriage muscles. It's a good idea to keep them strong.

A correctly "hovered" Plunge Pose will strengthen your abdominal muscles without creating excessive demand on your lower back—one of the potential issues of some traditional core exercises like sit-ups. It also helps stabilize healthy head position. It's a great pattern to develop, so once you've got it, take full breaths (every one is a rep) and maintain it as long as is comfortably available for you.

RELEASE

When you're done Plunge, relax your ankles and wrists. Make fists with fingers and toes, then splay them all widely. Draw circles in all directions with your feet and hands, stretching out your wrists. Take a couple of moments to honor hands and feet. We do a lot of work focusing on the center body and large muscle groups, but remember; this is really all one thing, your body. When we respect one part, we respect the whole thing.

Once you're through honoring your distal joints, just draw your knees toward your shoulders and put your palms on your kneecaps. Roll your skull side to side a bit, if it feels good. Relax and take a deep breath.

Don't worry. We'll do more hard stuff in just a second.

GOALS

- strengthen the front of the neck, particularly the scalenes, longus colli, and longus capitis
- develop stable core strength through breathing
- strengthen tissue around major joints in the arms and legs, compressing their respective joint capsules in a safe (unloaded) position
- open the back body gently

Once you're done with Plunge, hold your knees to your chest and rock and roll on your back a few times, then sit up.

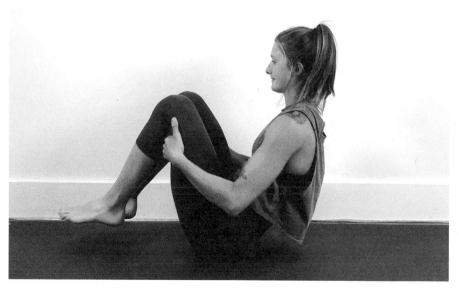

Rock and roll to bring yourself up to a seated position, then lie prone on your mat.

Back Strengthening Sequence

Cobra

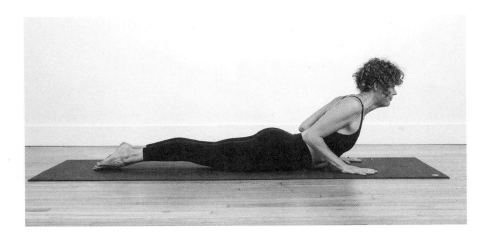

SETUP

Lie prone on your mat with your face smushed against the floor like a lamprey on a whale shark. (Notice how, with your face on the mat, your neck is in a relatively neutral position. If you were to lift your head and put your chin forward on the mat, which is intuitive for many of us, we are set up in hyperextension in the neck. Which we're trying to avoid.)

Put your hands flat to the ground right under your shoulders, so your elbows point upward. We don't have to be exact with the position here. Find a placement that feels comfortable in your shoulders and wrists.

Spread your fingers widely on the mat. I like to picture the widely splayed foot of a salamander, or a frog, or, you know, anything amphibious.

Get as much contact as you can between your hands and the mat, then put your legs together.[107]

ENTRANCE

Exhale: Press your thighs into the mat and draw your shoulder blades together on your back.

Inhale: Push your hands down and back, like you're trying to drive your mat backward, as you peel your heart up off the floor.

Avoid leading this posture with your eyeballs. Instead, try to maintain a neutral position in your neck and shoulders as you lift up. You'll probably notice your neck wants to grip (posterior chain trying to pull on your skull) and your shoulders want to round forward (upper back disengaging). This will often happen when you're trying to get Cobra to lift "way up" as high as you can. Take it easy; do what's available without losing the details.

ASSESSMENT

If we can hold the neck, shoulders, and pelvis in line during Cobra, we are in good shape. The difficulty here, of course, is that it is relatively easy in Cobra to create the *illusion* of "achievement" or "depth" by performing it mostly—and in some cases almost exclusively—in the most mobile portions of the spine; the cervical spine (the neck) and the thoracolumbar junction (where your rib cage meets your lower back).

Some of our assessment here can be visual: Are you jutting your chest and rib cage out? Is the back of your skull dropping into the back of the neck? You can also just feel for it. If you're compressed in the lower back or gripped in the back of your neck, you will know—you just have to feel for it.

Keep the magic points grounded.

---

[107] This "legs together" thing doesn't work perfectly for everyone. That's fine; find a narrow-ish width that works in your body.

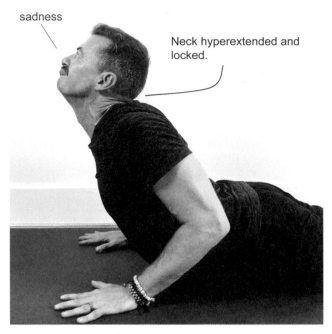

Chris has hyperextended his neck and is now sad.

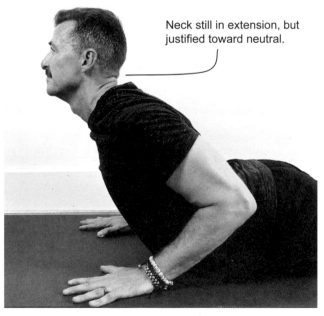

Chris has released excessive neck tension and is now really chill.

"MAGIC POINTS"

This is a bit of a Josephine. We are going to talk about how you place your hands on the mat, but in order to do that, we have to backtrack to your forearms.

You probably already know you've got two bones in your forearm, the radius and the ulna. If you hold your hand out in front of you like you're using a computer mouse, in pronation, your ulna is on the outside edge of your forearm. It is larger at the elbow and forms the majority of your forearm's connection to the humerus at the elbow. It is much smaller toward the hand, where it provides relatively weak support to the pinky side of your palm. Basically, your ulna provides a strong connection at the elbow and a (relatively) weak one at the hand. Cool?

OK, your radius does the opposite. It is relatively small at the elbow (which allows it to spin, or "radiate," around the joint, so your hand can pronate and supinate) and quite large and dense at your hand. So, the radius creates a weaker connection at the elbow and a stronger connection at the hand. Got it? Awesome.

We have two general lines of support, one from each bone in the forearm. They go:

1. Ulna—carpals—3rd and 4th metacarpals—phalanges of the pinky and ring fingers

2. Radius—carpals—1st and 2nd metacarpals—phalanges of the index and ring fingers

The ulna provides support to the ring and pinky fingers, but it's fairly weak. Notice the ulna-to-pinky-and-ring-finger connection here. There is no stable bone-to-bone joint between the ulna and these fingers, which has the benefit of increasing mobility in your hand. However, it means the pinky side of the human hand has much less support when under pressure. There's a structure there called the triangular fibrocartilage complex (TFCC, pictured here as an actual triangle, which it is not) that helps stabilize the connection between the ulna and the carpal bones. When your arms are extended and pronated—like in Downward Facing Dog—the TFCC is particularly vulnerable to injury. We don't want that. It's an important structure, so we try not to put excessive pressure directly on it for prolonged periods of time.

Since the line of your radius projects to the first and second metacarpals, these metacarpals have the most support, especially around the wrist. The short way of saying this is: The index side of your wrist is much stronger and steadier than the pinky side, primarily because of the way your forearm bones meet your hand bones. This is why, for example, boxers are taught to punch with their first two knuckles (index and middle) and not the last two.

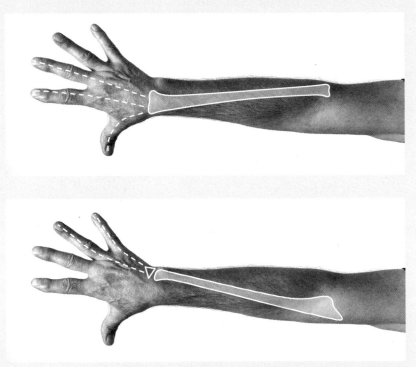

The radius provides primary support to the first two fingers and thumb.

If you punch with the last two knuckles you have much less stability and you're at much greater risk of breaking your hand.[108] These lines are not entirely distinct, they are bound together and integrated into one another in a holistic tension structure. However, in terms of bony support, they are somewhat independent.

Now look at your palm a moment. Right where your index finger connects with the body of your hand, there's a pad that's kind of like the ball of your foot.[109] It is where the first metacarpal meets the first phalange and the force of your radius is projected through to your fingers. It's what we like to call a "magic point."[110]

When you're doing work with your hands on the floor, we want to keep the magic points well-connected to the mat. This can help protect your wrists because we are intentionally using their strongest, most stable bony connection as the line of force. Conversely, if we ground through the *outside* of your hand, we are putting a great deal of weight on a fairly delicate area of the wrist with weak forearm support. This can

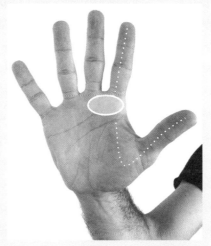

The magic point of the hand, with the L of the index finger and thumb.

---

[108] Least amount of risk? Don't punch people.

[109] This is called the first metacarpophalangeal joint. Palm readers call it the "Mound of Jupiter." It is approximately the same as the reflexology point for the heart line. For more information, please see your phone.

[110] Largely because going through that radius and ulna stuff every class is a total bore and everything is just simpler if you call it "magic!" and move on.

lead to issues in the wrists and shoulders, in particular, which is significant because the many common yoga injuries—along with hamstring pulls—involve the wrists and shoulders.

So, to recap: Due to the shape of your forearm bones, the index side of your wrist is much more stable and less prone to injury. We can use this design to our advantage while putting force through our hands into the mat. Focus on grounding through these magic points on your hands in poses like Dog, Plank, and Cobra.

- Notice if you're rolling the weight of the pose to the pinkie edge of your hands. Establish the magic points of the hands strongly, with the L of index finger and thumb as the most heavily grounded line on the hand.

- If your shoulders are gripped up in your neck, or they are diving forward of the line of the heart, back off a bit and reestablish their position. Cobra has the potential to make your upper back strong and keep you out of shoulder hunch, but only if we maintain the "strong upper back" pattern. Keep the shoulder blades glued to your back and your chest open.

BREATHING

In Cobra, and all the back bends away from the floor, there is a good amount of pressure on the torso. The weight of the body compresses the abdomen and creates resistance to deep breathing. We can use this to our advantage, if we so choose. Belly breathing here can strengthen the respiratory diaphragm. Chest breathing in Cobra has more potential to open the rib cage and shoulders, as the breath is more effectively confined to the upper torso.

Experiment with how you place the breath, using neutral position around the lower back–pelvis and the neck as a guide. Exhales can help establish lift and length in the spine, but that means taking full, intentional inhales to prepare.

OPTIONS

In time, if you like, you can begin to look up toward the ceiling. The key is that we keep from sinking into the back of the neck in a tight, gripped, hyperextended position. Instead, think about *lengthening* the neck into the back bend as you look up. This will require much more focus than just "look up," and you likely won't be able to look as high up toward the ceiling, but it will help you establish a healthy back-bending pattern.

If you have established a strong, generalized back bend, you might try to float your hands off the floor. This is a tough move: it greatly increases the load on your back muscles, which may make them start to grip up and localize the back bend. Likewise, your breath will probably become much more challenging. Remember, the overall pattern of the pose is much more important than any particular embellishment to it. Do what arrives within the pattern of the pose.

GOALS

- integrate and activate the posterior chain evenly
- strengthen the back, particularly the rhomboids and lats
- open the chest
- support spinal decompression

Crocodile

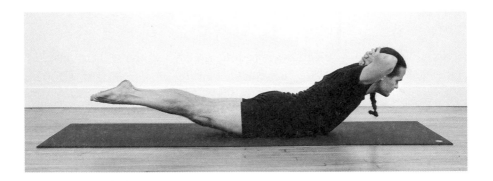

SETUP

Lie prone with your forehead down on the mat and legs together, then interlace your fingers behind your head. Make sure your hands are on the back of your skull, not the back of your neck.

Start with your elbows resting on either side of your head. Lift your elbows high off the mat, and bring your shoulder blades together on your back.

ENTRANCE

Lift your head and chest off the floor, driving your head back into your hands.

Once you've lifted your chest up, lift the legs up off the mat.

ASSESSMENT

I personally love Crocodile because it's so hard to cheat in the position. With your hands behind your head, you prevent your shoulders from rolling forward. Likewise, it's a bit more difficult to grip in the back of your neck because your hands prevent you from looking up too far.

- The primary way Crocodile can fall apart is around the elbows. You may find that once you start to lift off the floor, the elbows start to swing forward, wrapping your forearms around your ears. This happens in part because of weak or inactive upper back muscles, combined with tension in the chest. Focus on keeping your elbows as wide as is available. This will take a good degree of upper back strength and may prevent you from lifting very high, but that's OK. Keep your attention on the upper back getting stronger, and your heart opening in the back bend.

- Apply a bit of resistance here by gently pushing your hands into the back of your head. At the same time, resist this pressure by pushing your head back into your hands. Only do this as it's comfortable with your neck, and to the degree you can without dropping your elbows forward.

- Finally, and this is a personal favorite, try to pull your head off. (Don't worry, you can't actually do it. Though if you're working with a neck injury, definitely hold off on this one.) To perform this action, you've got to engage your lats and triceps, which helps stabilize your upper back while encouraging length in the spine.

BREATHING

Crocodile restricts the opening of the top of your chest by drawing the pectoral muscles toward their full length, which creates a line of tension across the upper ribs and collarbones. This, paired with the compression of the lower belly, can challenge your breathing.

Once you've assembled the pose, really home in on taking steady breaths as best you can. Crocodile is a pretty simple shape. It doesn't need much refinement once you have the basics, so take this opportunity to engage your breath with gentle intention. The intention is simply, "in and out, in and out." Holding the upper back stable while opening the chest will pattern your body toward Healthy Neutral in the posture.

OPTIONS

- If you're looking for more shoulder opening than back strength, you can practice Locust Pose with your hands clasped behind your back.

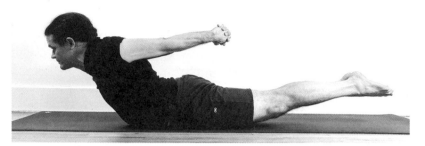

Locust Pose with the shoulder stretch.

◆ To add difficulty, bend your knees so your toes point to the ceiling. Make sure you keep your knees together and try to lift your thighs up in the pose. Go slowly, this one is a bear. (Or … you know … a crocodile.)

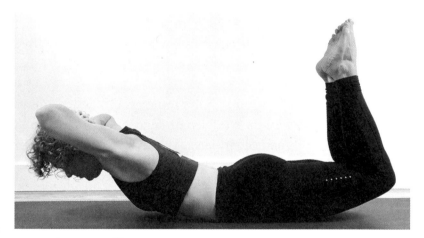

Intermediate Crocodile Pose.

GOALS

◆ develop posterior chain strength, particularly in the upper back, glutes, and hamstrings

◆ open the chest, especially the pectoral muscles

Bow

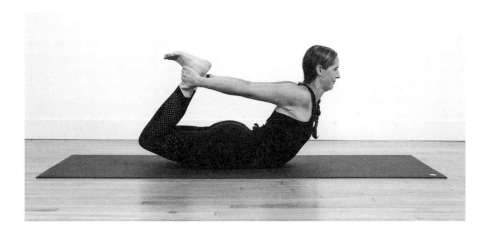

SETUP

Start prone with your forehead on the floor. Bend your knees and reach back to grab hold of your feet or your ankles. If you're taking hold of your ankles, dorsiflex your feet (bend your ankles) to stabilize your grip.

Before we get going, notice your grip. See if there's more pressure on the pinkie side edge of your hand, or the index finger side. See if you can firmly establish the pinky side. You might find it helps turn your shoulders back and open your chest. Maintain pressure there, and then reestablish the index side of your grip as well. Consider pressing into the magic points.

ENTRANCE

Kick back into your hands a bit, just enough to put tension into the chain of arms and legs. Feel this tension in the shoulders and gently let them draw back, opening the chest.

Inhale: Peel your chest up away from the floor.
Exhale: Keep lifting, drawing your shoulder blades together and down your back.

Lift your head to look forward, eyes on the horizon.

ASSESSMENT

Maintain focus on lifting with the muscles of the back and the flow of the breath. The kick is a secondary engine for this one; make sure you're not overdoing it. If you make the kick your main driver here, you may find that the back bend sinks into the neck and mid-back.

A good way to stabilize the pose is to focus on keeping the pelvis strongly grounded into the mat. You might notice that as you lift up. The weight of the body starts to press into the lower abdomen as the tailbone starts to float up in the back bend. If you can keep the tailbone "tucked" down toward the mat, you'll encourage greater integration and activation of the abdominal muscles, while avoiding the localized back bend.

BREATHING

Inhales open the chest, shoulder to shoulder. Exhales draw the ribs in.

Whatever you do, keep the breath moving, even if it's just a little bit. There's a very common tendency in Bow to lift up high, and then hold the breath and just try to ride the whole thing out by sitting on top of the pressure in the torso. Don't do that. It will be more challenging, but moving the breath in the posture will help strengthen the muscles of the core and back.

THE RULE OF THREE RIDES AGAIN

Remember that one of the best ways to support the spine in a back bend is to turn on the anti-back bend muscles. The forward "crunch" muscles will stabilize the torso and help keep the spine out of localized compression. In poses like Bow and Camel, think about allowing the exhales to draw the front of the rib cage down and in toward the spine while the top of the chest lifts and opens. These actions resist one another, which is, of course, the point.

OPTIONS

If you want to make this one harder, try to do it without lifting your thighs from the mat.

If you can't reach your feet or ankles behind you, use a strap. Completing the "circuit" of the posture—the full connection of feet to hips to shoulders to hands to feet—is important to the pattern, especially when it comes to opening your chest in the back bend.

GOALS

- ◆ open the front of the chest
- ◆ strengthen the quads and lower legs
- ◆ strengthen the muscles of the back
- ◆ decompress the spine within a back bend

Child's Pose

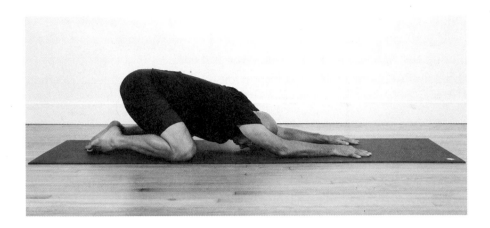

From prone on the mat, just press yourself back and put your hips on your heels. Knees wide. Arms forward or down alongside your body.

Let this one be easy. Relax your neck and feel the breath moving in your back.

If resting in Child's Pose is challenging for you, put a block or some support underneath your hips. If that doesn't make it better, just sit in a comfortable position for a few breaths.

Dog Sequence

Forearm Plank

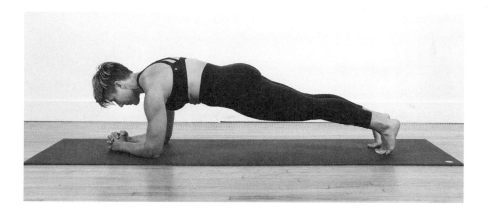

SETUP

Place your elbows on the mat directly under your shoulders and interlace your fingers in a two-handed fist.

Start with your knees on the mat, a little way back from the line of your hips, and tuck your toes to the mat.

Tuck your tailbone down and draw your ribs in tightly to your spine. We want to establish strong front-body engagement here, before we fully load the posture. If we don't, the core muscles may not be properly integrated, and the weight of the body will likely sink into the back of the spine.

At the outset, it will resemble Cat pose with the rounded position of the spine.

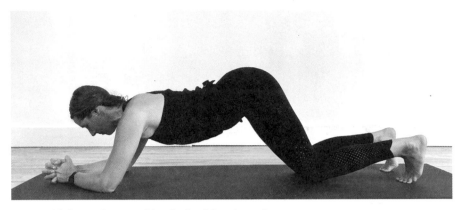

Start with knees down and let the back bend sag for a moment.

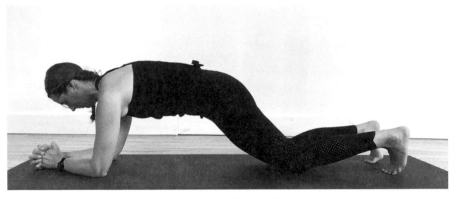

Exhale to draw the ribs in and turn on the abdominal wall.

ENTRANCE

Drive your heels back and lift your knees. Make your knees *almost* lock but not quite.

ASSESSMENT

Forearm Plank is a clinic on both Healthy Neutral and the challenge of avoiding habitual compensation patterns (cheats). If you've got cheats, you will find them hard to avoid in this position for very long.

Since the position is simple, we can keep the assessment pretty bare-bones:

- back of the neck long
- skull in line with the rest of the spine
- shoulders neutral (in the plane of the heart) or pressed slightly downward, so the upper back opens
- ribs in
- pelvis neutral

Some of these will fall into the "easy to say, hard to do" category. I find that setting the position of the skull and ramping the neck is the most challenging part of the pose for most students. If you find this is the case, save it for last. Do the other things first and then set the skull as best you can. Pay close attention to the way Forearm Plank arrives in your own body. It is often a great way to assess your personal patterns.

Also, it's almost universal for beginners to set their elbows too wide on the mat. My guess is something in the human lizard brain fundamentally understands that triangles are more stable (and thus need less muscular support) than rectangles. Though I don't think your lizard brain uses those words, per se. I imagine it slowly blinks four separate eyelids over a honey-colored iris with a pupil the shape of a pentagram. But the concepts are in there nonetheless. Set vertical support in the upper arms and be diligent about maintaining it. This forces your shoulder, chest, and back muscles to do most of the work of holding you up.

BREATHING

If we're holding Healthy Neutral, there will be a great deal of tension throughout the torso. If we maintain the structure of the pose, the breath will have difficulty localizing into one area. This is great. There's no need to push the breath around; just keep it moving and focus on holding your shape. If you can maintain neutral during Forearm Plank, moving the breath evenly throughout the torso, every breath becomes a rep to strengthen stable upright human posture.

OPTIONS

Most modifications here have to do with hand position. They're all fine as long as you don't lose the vertical line from elbows to shoulders.

* Palms to the mat, fingertips touching.

* Hold a block between your palms, thumbs up.

* Frame a block between the L shape of the index finger and thumb on either hand.

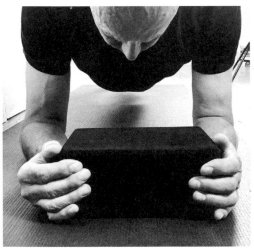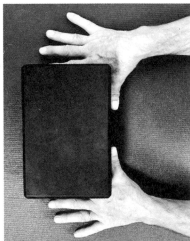

GOALS

* develop core strength

* integrate core strength with lower body support

* strengthen shoulders and arms

Dolphin

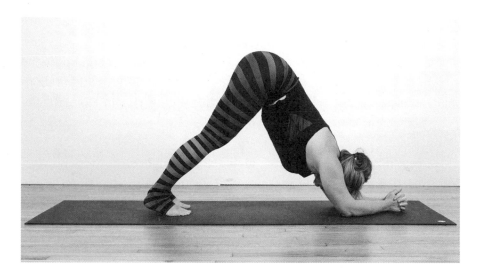

SETUP

Be in Forearm Plank.

ENTRANCE

Walk your feet toward your elbows until you're up on your toes with your hips high in the air.

Keep a slight bend in your knees.

ASSESSMENT

Notice again, the elbows might try to swing wide to make the A-frame support. Be disciplined and try to keep your elbows at about the width of your shoulders.

With the hips entering deep flexion, you'll most likely avoid any localized compression in the mid- or lower back. However, pay attention to hyperextension in the neck. If you find yourself gripping the muscles behind your skull, try to unlock there and find some space.

If the neck is gripped in hyperextension, one possibility is to engage other support structures to help distribute the load of the posture. Your arms, legs, and torso can all participate in supporting the posture. Try driving the balls of the feet back and the elbows down. Soften your jaw. Work on gently drawing the ribs back toward the spine to support the weight of the torso. Consider that when the arms and legs and abdominal muscles are not fully participating in holding you in Dolphin, the posterior chain, particularly in your neck, must work in overdrive to compensate.

Depending on your hamstring mobility, you might start to round your lower back as you move farther into the position. Take your time setting the posture. Don't be afraid to twerk a little, tilting the pelvis into flexion and extension gently a few times. Remember that Healthy Neutral beats depth every time. If you cannot maintain neutral, don't walk the pose in quite as far.

If you can maintain Healthy Neutral in the torso, especially in the pelvis, then you can explore straightening your legs further. The more you straighten your legs, the more you may start to "pull" on the pelvis and potentially move out of neutral. Experiment with this resistance and your ability to stabilize the pelvis as you straighten the legs and lengthen the hamstrings. (By contrast, it is possible to bend the knees *too much* and similarly tilt the pelvis out of neutral.) Be gentle with it. You're in a weird position and we want to avoid putting excessive strain on your lower back.

BREATHING

As in Forearm Plank, holding neutral in Dolphin requires a lot of focus. It's fine just to breathe normally the whole time. You might explore moving the inhales up toward the hips, and the exhales to press your hips back and up farther.

OPTIONS

Dolphin is an effective setup for Forearm Stand. If you have that in your practice, go for it. I'm not teaching that here, as instruction on inversions is only available in Premium Book, which requires a monthly subscription to my online life-coaching service and a nice little personalized note.[111] Or cake.

GOALS

- strengthen shoulders and triceps
- stabilize core
- open posterior chain
- pattern Healthy Neutral breathing in inverted position

---

[111] This joke is going to come back to haunt me in, like, seven years when I pull a hard pivot and go full Tim Robbins and write my *real* book, *Eternally Snowballing Income and Unassailable Happiness for Human Beings.* It's gonna rule.

Downward-Facing Dog

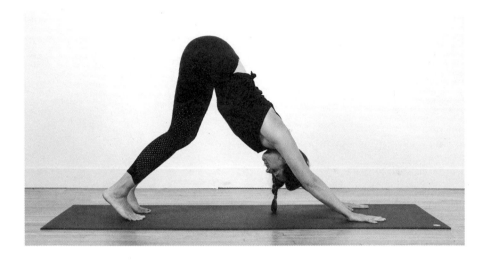

SETUP

Start in tabletop, with your hands directly under your shoulders and your knees under your hips. From there, walk your knees back a bit—maybe eight inches or whatever—and tuck your toes so they're on the mat. Spread your fingers widely for as much skin-to-mat contact as possible.

Draw your belly in to support your mid-spine and float your knees off the ground.

ENTRANCE

Inhale: Fill the back of your rib cage.
Exhale: Press your hands down to send your hips up and back.

Don't straighten your legs all the way to start. For most people, straightening your legs in a well-constructed Down Dog will not be available for some time, usually because of tension in the hamstrings, calves, and ankles. It's all right; work from Healthy Neutral in the torso to start and measure outward from there.

DOWN DOG IS NOT A RESTING POSE

You may have heard this before: Downward Facing Dog Pose is hard. It's arguable that, despite its presence in many beginner-level classes, it's an intermediate-level posture. I wouldn't mention this except it is also probably the most common pose in daily practice today, the pose people most associate with yoga in general, and is occasionally taught as a place to "rest" during a flow class. Personally, I don't think of Down Dog as a place to rest.

To do this pose well, you need strong shoulders and wrists, good core stability, powerful thighs and calves, a supple posterior chain, and well-developed awareness of your position in space while inverted. Almost every one of these traits is rare among true beginners. If we treat Down Dog like a rest position, it will likely put excessive strain on the mid-back, sink into the shoulders, "hang" on the tension in the hamstrings,[112] or some combination of the three.

As we mentioned back in the section on magic points, wrist and shoulder injuries are some of the most common among yoga students. When we simply rest in Down Dog, there are very good odds we aren't mindfully grounding our hands into the mat or engaging strength to create support and space in and around the shoulder joint. These seemingly minor concerns, stretched out over the course of a practice—sometimes years, sometimes a single class—can lead to injury, which, among other things, make people stop doing yoga. And when people stop doing yoga, a freak typhoon hits Isla Nublar and knocks the power grid offline and, well … you know the rest …[113]

---

[112] In which case the hamstrings are at their maximum length, so they're tight like ropes. At that point you can just rest into this tension like grandad in a hammock.

[113] Hang onto your butts.

ASSESSMENT

Like Forearm Plank and Dolphin, focus on keeping your spine in Healthy Neutral. This may limit your access to "depth" in the pose, but that's fine. You might not get your head between your arms all the way, or your heels down, or your legs straight. This is all fine. Work from a place of stability in the center body and go from there.

Keep the magic points grounded.

BREATHING

Same as the last two. Practice maintaining Healthy Neutral instead of back bend breathing. Mindfully engage the abdominal wall in the exhales.

OPTIONS

If this hurts your wrists or shoulders in any way, if it pulls on anything in a way that makes you uncomfortable, sit it out.

GOALS

- strengthen core muscles, shoulders, and hips
- strengthen the legs
- open the posterior chain, particularly in the legs
- open the front of the chest and shoulders
- decompress the spine

Pigeon

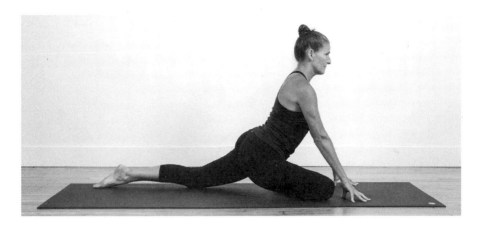

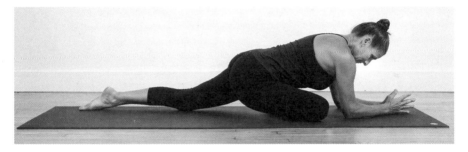

SETUP

From Down Dog, lift your right leg high behind you (Three-Legged Dog) then bend your right knee and open your hips to the right (a.k.a. Fire Hydrant Pose, if you're gross). Take a breath here.

As you exhale, smoothly swing your right knee forward. Try to touch your hairline to your kneecap and feel your core engage strongly. Nice and easy from here, let your right knee come down near your right wrist. Set your right shin at a 45-degree (ish) angle relative to the front of your mat.

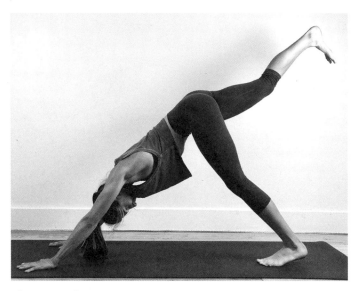

Three-Legged Dog.

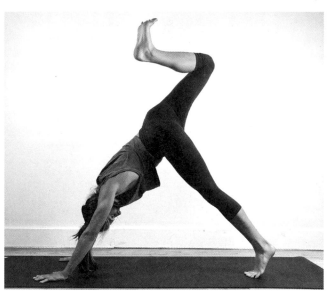

Scorpion Kick, a.k.a. "Fire Hydrant Pose" (ew).

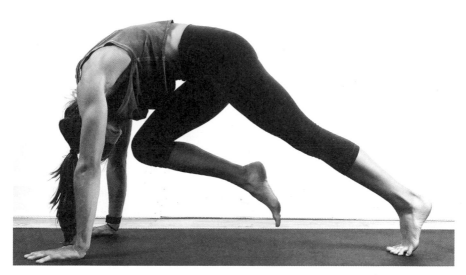

Knee to nose over Plank.

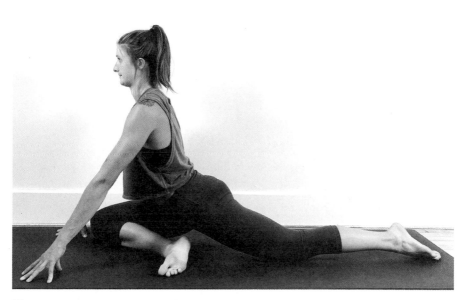

Pigeon.

ENTRANCE

Draw your belly in. Inhale and push your hands down, lifting your chest up. Exhale and gently lean forward, drawing your heart forward to keep your spine long.

If it's available, go down to your elbows. If not, bring your heart forward and down to the degree you can.

ASSESSMENT

At least in Foundations, let's avoid "Roadkill Pigeon," where you just flop on the ground across your right shin. Even if it's like, "Ah-h-h, man, but I get this really *juicy stretch* when I just collapse like a tranquilized honey badger and I *re-e-ally like it.*"

This is an important moment. Stop the music. Put down your phone. (No, seriously, put your phone in the nearest pair of Doc Martins you can find. Or whatever.)

I want you to hear me on this one: Stretching pain is not good.

Pause

Again: Stretching pain is not good.

STRETCHING PAIN IS NOT GOOD

You OK? Still with me? Maybe you're flipping the book over and squinting angrily at the publisher's seal and going "Who in the *world*" and getting your phone out of that boot and googling who in their right mind would allow such content into the world.[114]

Bear with me just a second. Hear what I'm not saying, here. I am not saying stretching pain is bad. I'm saying stretching pain is not good. As in, it is not *always* good. As in, it is not *inherently* good.

---

[114] "I mean, I could take the flippant sarcasm and the so-pleased-with-yourself tone and the jokes-as-footnotes gimmick up until now, but this? This is a bridge too far!"

When you started yoga, you may have had an experience like mine: I was stiff and creaky and my body didn't move the way I wanted it to. Then the teacher told me to do some kind of stretch, something I would never normally do, and I came up against this wall of pain. And at first, I found it deeply uncomfortable. But I knew that yoga was supposed to be good for me and the teacher was so nice and calm and confident and everyone around me was doing the stretch and they seemed so happy and screaming bloody murder would have really disrupted the vibe in the room. (I think those were milk- and vetiver-scented candles?) So I stayed in the pose. And over time I got used to it. And I felt great after class.

I kept coming to my practice, and in time I created a new attitude toward that stretching pain; it didn't actually *hurt*. Not for me. Not anymore. For me stretching pain had become a beautiful sensation, a feeling of vitality from the darkness within, like the glow of phosphorescent algae on a starlit beach. It took on an almost religious significance, this pain. I sought it. I desired it. If I'm being honest, I still often do.

Sound familiar, maybe? In my experience this is a very common narrative among yoga students. And it isn't necessarily bad. Stretching is useful. Mobility is useful. These things are a vital part of maintaining a healthy body.

But stretching and healthy mobility aren't the only things happening in this little yoga story. In this story we also have a process called reframing, whereby I mentally redefined the way I felt about stretching pain. I changed my mind. What used to cause me suffering became, with practice, something I pursued or even enjoyed. How? I practiced an attitude—an idea—repeatedly, until it made my brain a different shape. Literally, that's what happened. I had something like "stretching pain sucks" patterns in my brain at first, then over time I remolded them into "stretching pain is fantastic" patterns. This process helped me first endure and then crave the work of developing mobility. It also created an impression in my mind, a higher-order pattern in the realm of belief beyond simple desire, that said something like, "Stretching pain is a sign I am getting healthier."

But this belief isn't actually true. I mean, it is usually true that the process of becoming healthier or more functional in your body will include stretching pain, but the assertion that stretching pain is *always* a sign of getting "better" or "healthier"? That's not really the case.

When you do a stretch, the pain you feel does not have an inherent value.[115] Stretching pain is simply a signal telling you that a muscle is close to its capacity, in terms of length, and that you might want to proceed carefully from there. It is a warning. It's not good or bad; it's value-neutral information. It says, "Hey, don't move too quickly past this point or we might sustain an injury."

Now, if we are trying to increase our range of motion, then this stretching pain is a sign we're heading in the right direction. Mindfully maintaining a stretch is how we increase the length of a certain muscle group. And for many beginners, this is a great goal. We want to be flexible enough to smoothly coordinate functional movement without undue resistance. Being too stiff is potentially problematic. Male athletes in particular can reduce their injury risk by stretching regularly. (However, there's evidence that most female athletes are already flexible enough and get no functional benefit from adding stretching to their routines.)

But what if we *don't* want to increase range of motion? What if we're mobile enough already and making the tissue looser will make our bodies less functional? There is no sensation for "You are making yourself unstable or hypermobile."[116] All we have is the warning signal of stretching pain.

This is particularly important with regard to hip openers, like Pigeon.

See, you really need stable hips. Like, really, really need them. Mobility in your hips is highly functional, for sure, but stability is equally essential

---

[115] We could make a very compelling argument that no sensations have inherent value, but I'm already too deep in this Bog of Eternal Stench to try to wade that Swamp of Sadness at the same time.

[116] Because, frankly, there isn't much use for this kind of signal. The concept of an organism spending precious time and energy to increase their range of motion outside of their basic needs is—in terms of evolution—sort of absurd.

to healthy movement. Especially in the long term. If you remove too much tension out of the soft tissue in and around your hips, you may alter the way your hips carry the weight of your upper body when you walk. When your foot hits the ground with each step, the tension of your connective tissue helps distribute the force of impact throughout your body. If you don't have enough tension in these tissues (or if you have too much), your body is less effective as a shock absorber. This is less of an issue if we're young; our bodies have relatively little wear on them and we are quite good at developing muscle strength to support our movements.[117] But as we get older, it becomes more difficult to develop and maintain muscle tone.

It's potentially problematic to have very little tension in the connective tissue around and throughout the pelvis as we age. Regardless of our fitness level, over time the little shocks of moving around in the world add up. Our joints take a beating through the course of human life, especially those in the lower body. It's wise to give them all the help we can provide.

It's also useful to note that your hips are complex joints. Your glutes alone are densely layered, arranged in myriad angles, and partitioned into multiple subgroups. If you go looking for stretching sensations somewhere in that dense weave of muscle and connective tissue, you'll probably find something. But just because you find a dragon doesn't mean you have to kill it. Some dragons eat alligators, and the alligators are seriously overpopulated on this particular fantastic delta/useless digression.

---

[117] Although there is some evidence that hypermobile people are more susceptible to chronic fatigue, as muscle activation requires energy. The theory goes: if you rely more on your muscles to absorb and distribute shock and less on your connective tissue, you use more energy. So when you move, you're constantly draining energy you might use elsewhere.

The second big issue with hip openers has to do with your hip labrum, a doughnut-shaped layer of cartilage inside your hip socket.[118] This cartilage prevents the ball of your femur from grinding against the wall of the acetabulum. The tricky part, though, is that cartilage does not have sensory nerves. So your labrum cannot, in the general sense, feel anything. If it becomes damaged, it cannot communicate with your brain to tell you there's something wrong.

If you put repeated and intense pressure on a particular part of your labrum by, say, driving the head of the femur into it at an odd angle, you can wear it down. And you will not even feel it happening. In fact, there's evidence that professional dancers with extreme hip mobility are more likely to develop osteoarthritis in their hips than the general population, as studies have shown that "repetitive extreme movements can cause femoral head subluxations and femoroacetabular abutments in female ballet dancers with normal hip morphologic features, which could result in early OA."[119] Basically, in extreme hip movements you may slightly dislocate your hip joint, and your thigh bone wears down your labrum like basil in a mortar and pestle.

You may now be thinking at this point that evolution really messed up here. If the hip is so important, and the labrum doesn't have nerves, why doesn't your body have some other signal to tell if you're doing something dangerous? One answer is that prehistoric human beings probably didn't need extreme hip mobility feedback. There's not much of a survival benefit to standing, sitting, or lying down with a leg behind your head. However, there is a pretty obvious survival risk: if a leopard rushes you and you're standing up on one leg with the other tucked behind your skull, you're ... well your chances of survival are diminished, let's say that.

---

[118] Acetabulum.

[119] Victoria B. Duthon, Caecilia Charbonnier, Frank C. Kolo, Elia Coppens, Pierre Hoffmeyer, and Jacques Menetrey, "Correlation of Clinical and Magnetic Resonance Imaging Findings in Hips of Elite Female Ballet Dancers," *Journal of Arthroscopy and Related Surgery* 29:3 (March 2013), 411–19, doi:10.1016/j.arthro.2012.10.012.

And the other answer, of course, is that you do have a feedback mechanism: your independent intelligence. Because the thing is, you don't have to believe what I'm saying here any more than you have to believe "stretching pain is always good." You can choose. I hope you choose my perspective, because I believe it will serve you better in the long term. But it's your call. You have the capacity to assess your practice with attention and information. You can set standards of your own and divine your own goals. You can determine what you think is functional, asking questions like, "What range of motion is useful for me in my life?" and "Do I need less tension in my hips, or more?"

If you can't tell already, this one is personal for me. I spent a lot of time and effort becoming exceptionally flexible through yoga practice. My yoga community complimented me on my extreme range of motion, and that validation drove me to further flexibility practice. I eventually was able to place both of my feet behind my head in Yoginidrasana, and I was proud of what I had accomplished. But shortly afterward my hips started to grind. When I walked my dog, I felt popping and clicking deep inside the joints. I soon discovered I could "crack" my hip joints like knuckles, almost at will.

The question I had to ask myself eventually was, "What's the point of putting my legs behind my head?" And if I took away Instagram likes and social validation and feeling like some kind of yoga god? If I just looked at the physical value? I couldn't come up with a decent answer.

What I sincerely hope is that we can honestly attend to our assumptions about what is helpful and useful and what is not. Again, you get to make your own choices based on your own priorities. As it turns out, "Roadkill Pigeon" is a really good pose for some people; it might do wonders for your body and your healing process. I only ask that you carefully consider your priorities before you chase extreme poses. You may find that some serve you and others just don't. But you'll never know until you ask.

BREATHING

Send your breath to the right hip, nice and easy.

OPTIONS

- ◆ If you happen to be one of these people who is already very open in the hips, try lifting the pose up from the floor a bit; perhaps eight to twelve inches off the mat. Gently square your hips forward and be mindful of your knees. We're putting additional load on the muscles by lifting the pose up. Take your time. In this format, Pigeon Pose is more of a strength position than a stretch one, which is an effective counterbalance for highly mobile hips.

- ◆ In time, you can make this lifted Pigeon more challenging by taking your hands off the ground.

- ◆ If you're still working on mobility, and getting your hands or elbows down safely doesn't feel available, you can use blocks for extra support.

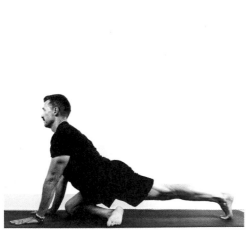
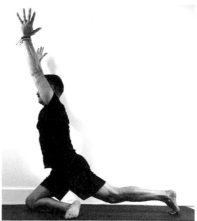

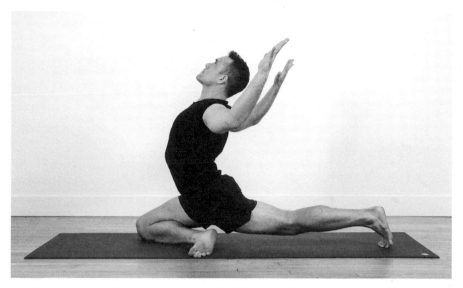

Breaking my own rules, here. Pretty localized back bend going on. Do as I say, not as I do, yeah?

GOALS

- open (and/or strengthen) the right hip
- lengthen the left hip flexor
- gently open the lower back

EXIT

"Pigeon Push-Up": Place your hands on the floor and tuck the toes of your back foot to the mat. Pull your belly in and push off the ground, keeping your right knee as close to your chest as possible.

Then swing your right leg back and up, into Three-Legged Dog. Shake out your leg then return to Down Dog.

Kneeling Sequence

Supine Warrior

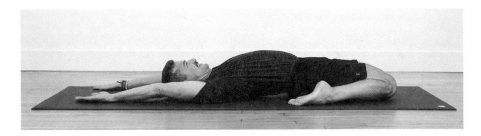

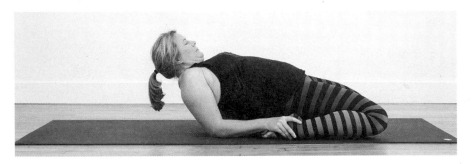

SETUP

Kneel to your mat with your knees close and your feet separate. You should have enough space between your feet to get your hips to the mat, but not more. Sit your hips down between your feet. You can sit on a block if that's better for you.

Hook your thumbs across the arches of your feet and roll your shoulders back. Tuck your chin toward your chest a bit.

ENTRANCE

Slowly lean back. If you can get your elbows to the floor, go there. If you can't, all good. Do what's available for you. Be mindful of your knees; make sure you're not pushing into or through any pain.

Keep your chin to your chest and look toward your navel through the whole entrance.

If you're on your elbows, you might explore taking the back of your rib cage down to the mat. Then your head.

ASSESSMENT

- Tone your navel to your spine and think about tucking your tailbone toward the front of your mat.

- You might feel the urge to let your head drop back. Try to avoid that urge. Instead, think about gently lengthening your spine as you lean back in the position. If your shoulders or the back of your ribcage land to the mat, then you can rest your head to the floor.

- Knit your ribs toward your spine; resist the impulse to make the posture back-bend deeply. The closer we can move the torso toward Healthy Neutral, the more we will open the front of the legs (particularly the quadriceps.)

BREATHING

Inhale to your back.
Exhale to knit the ribs and tuck the tail.

OPTIONS

- Sit on a block if it feels better on your knees.

- If you can get your back down to the floor, reach your arms straight upward toward the ceiling and present a beach ball to God. Feel your upper back rounding down toward the mat and breathe deeply.

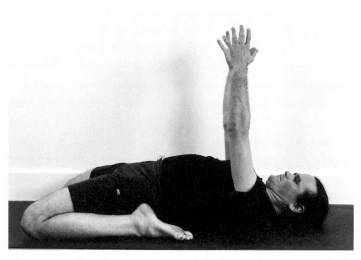

The "arms up" option allows you to knit the ribs down more effectively.

◆ If you're very mobile and want to activate the pose, reach your arms straight back alongside your ears toward the back of the mat, palms up (pictured). Imagine you have a small (maybe six or seven months old) rhinoceros sitting on your hands. Remember for a moment that this is a heavy, somewhat temperamental species. The mother is likely nearby. So no fighting. You can't move your hands.

◆ As you exhale, knit your ribs and try to lift the rhino. Remember, it ain't going anywhere. The idea is to create internal resistance in the position as you breathe. This action will increase the tension across your quads, so go mindfully and do not put excessive pressure on your knees.

GOALS

◆ open quadriceps and hip flexors

◆ open the fronts of the ankles

◆ decompress the spine

◆ strengthen diaphragmatic breathing

◆ open the chest (with arms overhead along the floor)

Half Tortoise

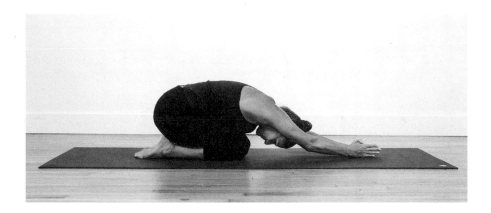

SETUP

Kneel on the mat with your hips on your heels and your knees together.

ENTRANCE

Inhale to take your arms overhead.
Exhale to lower your upper body down along your legs. Gently stretch your arms forward along the mat with your palms together.

ASSESSMENT

Don't work too hard. Seriously. The forward curve of your thoracic spine (lordosis) is laid against your thighs here. The upward resistance from your thighs will gently flatten out this lordotic curve and create space in the posterior spine as you breathe. We don't want to put too much effort into this. Instead, we focus on relaxing into it. Let gravity into the position. Explore the capacity of your spine to lengthen through the pulse of the breath.

BREATHING

Breathe gently into your back. Imagine the ocean waves—the deep ocean—moving gently along the muscles of your back. Or you might visualize the large sheet of muscle across your back as the outer tissue of a single lung; let that one unified structure pulse with the breath.

OPTIONS

You can adjust your hand position to address different tension patterns around the neck and shoulders. Some favorites of ours:

◆ Gently open your hands like a book so the palms face upward. Make sure the book is family-friendly and not Harry Potter of any kind.[120]

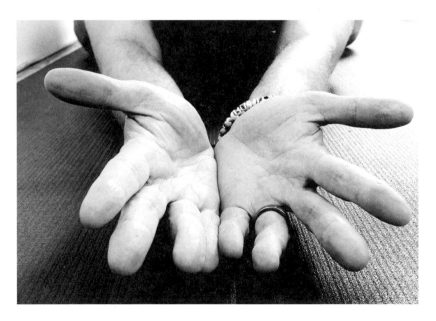

◆ With palms together, bend your elbows to put your hands behind your head. Let the position gently open the triceps.

---

[120] Don't @ me; I've never read them.

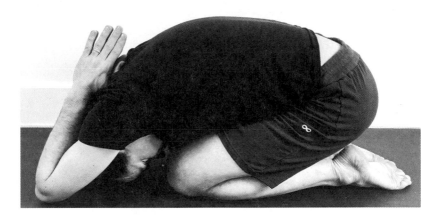

◆ Place your fingertips down firmly on the mat, like you're protecting two precious limes.[121] With your fingertips, push down on the mat and pull gently on the floor.

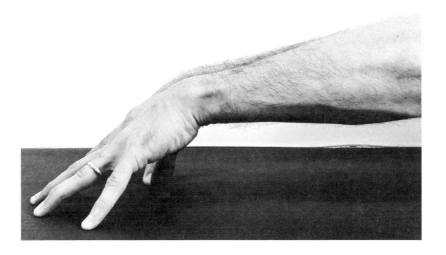

---

[121] Maybe the limes have the directions to the Ark of the Covenant on them and you can only get there and open the Spirit Vault by following the inscriptions on their rinds. And Tom Hanks is obviously there, but he's pushing his eyebrows together and not doing any physical comedy, so the mood is clearly solemn and it's obviously important to protect these limes.

Camel

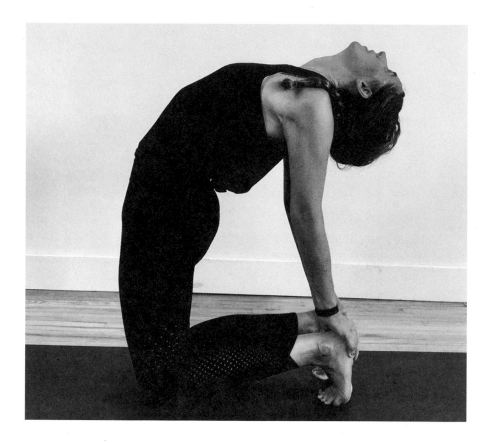

SETUP

From kneeling, set your knees at hip width and tuck your toes to the mat.

Sit back on your heels and put your hands behind your hips. Fingers down toward your butt.

If it's available to you, drive your hips forward first to lift up (instead of leading with your shoulders). Go easy.

Once you're up, use your fingers to drive your glutes down, helping you tuck your tailbone. Draw your belly in and up, and roll your shoulders back. For now, keep your chin close to your chest.

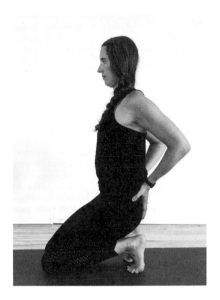 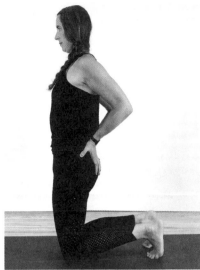

ENTRANCE

Inhale to lift and open your chest.

Exhale to lean back gently, opening your heart toward the ceiling above you.

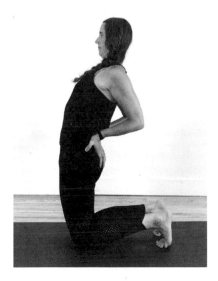

ASSESSMENT

Camel is a wonderful back bend, and a challenging one. It can teach us a great deal about our approach to the practice. The biggest consideration, I think, is the way we measure success in the position.

If you're measuring success in Camel with the question, "How far can I go back?" then you will likely sink the pose into localized compression without adequate core support. You can most likely bend farther if you sink into your joints, so if your goal is greater bending of the body, you might lose muscular support in the position.

If you're measuring success by asking, "How high can I get my heart center?" then you have a much better shot at activating core support to lengthen the spine and open the muscles of the chest. Upward action—lift—requires muscle activation to resist gravity. You've got to turn something on to make the posture move *upward*. Do that. Lift, and feel how the muscles of the torso support you.

A nickname for Camel is "Tractor Beam Pose." Imagine that the aliens have arrived and they want to take you home to your people.[122] Like all tractor beams, it holds you by your chest and pulls you upward from there. Feel the tractor beam pulling you up, taking you to Interstellar Burning Man, opening your heart toward the sky.

BREATHING

Inhale to open the chest.
Exhale to tuck the tailbone and knit the ribs.

OPTIONS

If you're well supported (read: not sinking into localized compression in your back) and can reach, you might try taking your heels in your hands. Let your shoulders open outward and grip strongly with your pinkie fingers.

You can explore gently letting your head fall back. Don't overdo this; just make it a nice, gentle, pillowy fall.

---

[122] You always knew you were a little weird for Earth, didn't you?

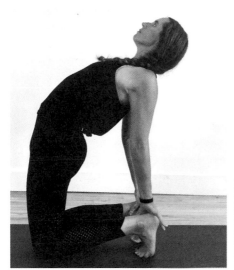 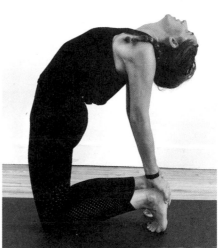

Wild Child

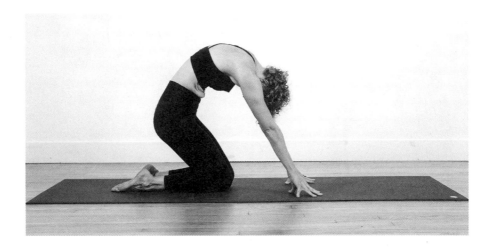

SETUP

From kneeling with knees together, put your hands to the mat about a foot beyond your knees. Lift up onto your fingertips.

Float forward a bit to bring your hips up off your heels.

ENTRANCE

Treat this like a standard Cat-Cow. Inhale to look upward, open the chest, and gently back bend.

As you exhale, round inward. Follow this progression: tuck your tailbone; lift your navel; knit your ribs; press your fingertips down to open your upper back; finally, slowly tuck your chin.

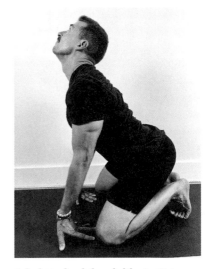

Inhale to back-bend, like in Cat-Cow. Note that in this image, Chris has his hands and feet set up in the "Screaming Child" variation, discussed in the Options section below.

Remember, often the default approach is to lead with your head and let the rest of the spine follow. Do the opposite: start at your tailbone and methodically work your way up the spine.

ASSESSMENT

Use the position to explore the relationship between abdominal activation and opening in the muscles of the back. If you work on pulling the front ribs and belly back toward the spine, you increase the pressure, and therefore the tension, on the back body. Explore this slowly. Look for subtlety and detail in your sensation, not necessarily depth or "progress." The shape of the pose is meant to keep you stable and safe in deep spinal flexion, an action that, when loaded, can put strain on your lower back. Here we have the support of both arms and legs as we engage the release of the back body.

Depending on your personal tension patterns, this may target different points at the back of the spine. For some people the opening will arrive lower in the back; for others, higher. You get the idea. Let it be personal. Let it inform you about your own body.

To explore further, you might change the distance between your hands and your knees. Generally, the farther away you walk your hands, the lower the opening moves on your back. If your hands are right next to your knees, you're more likely to direct the opening in the upper back, between the shoulder blades. Explore gently.

In time, you might occasionally work a "general" approach; try to evenly distribute the opening sensation throughout the entire back.

BREATHING

Imagine the muscles of your back as a single sail. (Let's say it's a jib. I like the cut of your jib.) Think of the inhales as a steady gust of wind that fills the sail, stretching it outward in all directions. On the exhales, practice front-body engagement. You can be general or detailed with these exhales, focusing on the whole torso or just one particular location; just use intention and focus.

OPTIONS

- ◆ As with all kneeling positions, feel free to sit on something if your knees need relief. You can also do Wild Child in a chair, sitting on the front edge of the seat with your feet flat on the floor and your hands on your knees. The object is to stabilize your hips. We don't need to chase any specific leg position.

- ◆ We do a thing we call "Screaming Child" sometimes, so called because it combines Wild Child with Toe Screamers. It goes like this: take your knees wide and tuck your toes to the mat, then sit on your heels. It will probably feel intense on the bottoms of your feet. Don't hurt yourself, but don't run away from the pain here either.[123]

Set your hands just forward of your knees, then spin your hands so your palms are facing forward and your fingers are pointing toward you on the mat. We're looking for an opening in the hands and wrists here. Again, don't push too hard, but don't sprint from the pain either. Once you've set that up, do your Cat-Cow entrance like in standard Wild Child. Adjust the pose as necessary to accommodate your wrists and feet.

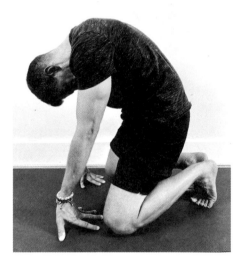

Screaming Child.

---

[123] We have an Aikido studio across the hall from our space in Vermont. They recently informed me that this position—sitting on your heels with your toes tucked underneath—is part of something they call "pain compliance," where you train yourself to endure, or breathe through, or mind-over-matter yourself past intense pain. The moral of the story, as always, is don't fuck with martial artists.

A PAUSE

After Wild Child, take a moment to just sit. Have your spine upright and shoulders relaxed. If sitting in the kneeling position is not comfortable for you, it's fine to sit cross-legged or place a block under your butt.

Place your dominant hand in your lap, palm up. Then place your other hand on top of it, palm up. Let your thumbs touch gently in Cosmic Mudra.

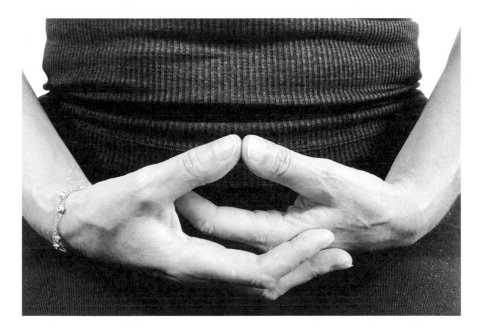

Look down at your mat and gently drop your chin. I'll invite you here to close your eyes.

Give yourself a few moments like this, exploring the interior darkness.

JOSEPHINE: STILLNESS IS NOT ONLY SELF-CARE

In the kneeling position, we might consider how deeply intertwined the components of the body are. Recall that when you move around the world, your legs are a vital part of your breathing system; they inform the tension in your hips and pelvis, which in turn manipulates the tension patterns through the lower back and abdomen, which in turn influences the rib cage and shoulders ... and your breathing influences the movement of your legs just the same. The system is integrated. Influence flows both ways.

We might also notice how our physical position is intertwined with our context in space and time. You are here, in this meditative position, because you are in this place in a yoga sequence. You are in this yoga sequence (presumably) because of an interest in yoga in general, which is pretty new in the Western world and has deep ties to colonialism and fitness fads dating back to the 1920s and the long-standing tradition of American-style magical thinking. This moment, in a sense, contains history. Not just *a* history but *all* history.

Consider perhaps that stillness and removal are not the same. You can investigate this within your body right now: the inactivity of your legs—putting no motor demand on your hip flexors or abdominal muscles—is itself a form of influence. Likewise, we see this in social interaction. Perhaps you have a friend who doesn't like to talk much in group settings, but somehow things are always different when they're in the room. Or maybe you've noticed that simply having your cell phone in your field of vision can cause you great distraction.

Presence—*existence*—has its own force. Invite the idea that while stillness is possible, non-influence is a delusion.[124] That you are a body with arms and legs means that you bear their influence at all times. That you are a person in space, even when you're alone, means you affect the world.

---

[124] Or, as Canadian prog-rock super-trio Rush once put it, "If you choose not to decide, you still have made a choice."

Now entertain one more idea: stillness is not only self-care. It is a way of shaping our connection with the world. Just as relaxation in one part of your body changes things elsewhere, so it goes for the larger systems of humanity: family, society, culture, civilization. Serenity and equanimity change a room just like passion does. When we are quiet, when we pause, we are not simply resting ourselves; we are informing our environment. And at the same time, we are allowing the room to change us right back.

This does not make stillness or relaxation better than action. But stillness is influential, like all behavior. Silence changes things. There is no manner of being that is disconnected from the whole, not in this life. We might entertain the notion that everything we do vibrates within and throughout an eternal and infinite network of shared information: a tapestry, if you will. In a way, yoga practice might, just might, be the work of owning this reality, along with all that it entails. Powerlessness and ultimate responsibility both move within this perspective, without resolution.

Closing Sequence

Staff Pose

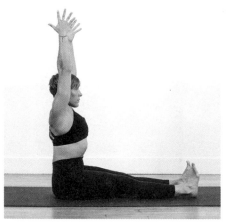 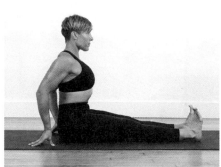

SETUP

Sit with your legs straight forward and your torso upright. If doing both isn't available, favor setting a neutral, upright position in your torso. Sit on a block, if necessary. Slightly bend your knees to engage your hamstrings, dorsiflex your ankles, and gently drive your heels into the mat. (We're just turning your legs on, for the most part.)

Place your hands behind you, perhaps on fingertips. Have a little bend in your elbows so your shoulders can move easily. Open your chest and sit tall.

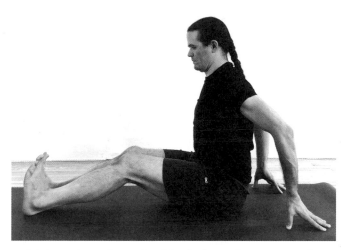

Isaiah is putting a deeper bend in the knees than most people need, for illustrative purposes. Communication skills.

ENTRANCE

If you can maintain upright posture in the torso, lift your arms overhead and reach for the sky.

ASSESSMENT

A teacher of mine used to say Staff is the hardest pose in all of yoga. I really like this sentiment because Staff doesn't look like a "hard" pose. It's not upside down or hypermobile or balancing on one foot or anything like that. It's just ... sitting on the floor. At first glance, we might think it should be easy.

But doing Staff *well* is surprisingly difficult, especially if you're going to be in it for any significant amount of time. This is partially because, for many students, Staff encourages a "slouch" in the mid-back when the legs are forward. Integrating the core strength to keep your spine upright with legs forward can require a considerable amount of effort. Breathing at the same time just makes it more challenging.

CORE SUPPORT BREATHING[125]

There are many interesting and beneficial ways to explore the breath during yoga practice, but if I had to pick a favorite, it would probably be Core Support Breathing. It illuminates how breathwork can be powerful and difficult, how the movement of air is a deeply muscular activity, and, when you start to get it, how breath helps create core stability that supports the structural work of the spine. It's great.

We do it like this. Sit upright in Staff Pose. If you need to make adjustments to the position (bending the knees, sitting on a block, etc.), go for it, and if upright posture isn't available in Staff Pose, try sitting in a chair.

Now lift your arms up overhead, about 30 degrees away from vertical. (If you try to get full vertical, you may start to back-bend and lose the upright position in the torso, so keep it within range.) Ground your heels and soften your jaw.

As you inhale, feel your rib cage expanding all the way around. Front and back. Try to get taller.

As you exhale, feel the corset of core strength gathering around the lower half of your torso. Front and back. Try to get taller.

Do this a few times, thinking: *Inhale to get taller, Exhale to get taller.* If you're really into it, it'll take a good deal of focus and strength. Good.

Notice how powerful you can make the breath. Notice how much work and how much motion is available to you just through this process. Notice how, in time, the simple act of breathing can in fact make you taller, decompressing your spine.

---

[125] This is based on a practice called Spinal Decompression Breathing that I picked up from Foundation Training (no relation), which is a therapeutic fitness program that I greatly admire. For our purposes, Core Support Breathing has mostly to do with the intention and engagement of the breath. In Foundation Training (I promise I found out about them after I named this yoga style) Spinal Decompression Breathing has many additional details added. It is a complete practice by itself. I recommend checking it out (https://youtu.be/lbNI4-vJSHQ).

BREATHING

Perform Core Support Breathing.

OPTIONS

As mentioned before, use a block to sit on if that helps you get more upright in the torso.

GOALS

- develop core stability and strength
- develop back strength
- pattern empowered breathing in Healthy Neutral
- integrate connection between leg and hip strength with core and back strength

Intense West Stretch

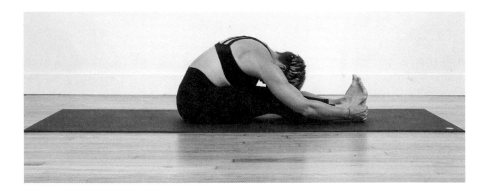

SETUP

Be in Staff Pose.

ENTRANCE

Inhale: Get tall.
Exhale: Gently reach forward to take hold of your toes. Hold them, but don't pull.

BREATHING

Gently let the breath massage the spine.

ASSESSMENT

Gently let the head fall and release the AO joint as best you can. This might take a couple of seconds. You'll likely discover a few sequential "layers" of tension there that have to be mindfully relaxed over time.

Give the pose a "hug."

ON HAMSTRINGS AND "HUGS" IN YOGA POSES

In the work of repatterning, we sometimes approach postures with the idea that they don't need to really "go" anywhere. Sometimes they don't have to develop into a different shape; they can just stay as they are. In certain poses like, say, Child's Pose, this is pretty obvious. This sort of forward fold can be practiced with similar softness.

As we have discussed before, opening the posterior chain is an admirable pursuit. Whether it's hamstrings, lower backs, necks, feet, etc., most people have one or more zones in the chain that could benefit from developing mobility and stability. However, if you stick around the yoga world long enough, you'll encounter an astonishing number of students with nagging hamstring injuries. (Should the two of us ever meet in person, dear reader, I will be among them.) I have a few theories about how this became the case.

1. We have a weird cultural standard for flexibility that is essentially framed around the question, "Can you touch your toes?" If you can touch your toes easily, then you're labeled as part of the decent-to-good flexibility group. If not, you're in the "Can't even touch my toes" group. It's an odd binary and that makes hamstring flexibility a little too central in the discussion of overall mobility.

2. A stretch to the hamstrings is relatively easy to find. All you have to do is lean or fall forward and there it is, loud and clear.

3. Most common hamstring stretches involve either gravity, leverage (meaning you have something to hold onto and then pull on), or both.

What we get out of all of this is a general tendency to chase hamstring stretches with ... let's call it "zeal." Zeal, plus gravity, plus leverage can be a recipe for injury.

Luckily, we can still practice mindful hamstring stretches within the greater work of posterior chain opening, and still keep ourselves safe. One way to do this is to turn on what we like to call a "hug" for the pose.

Embrace the posture with a comfortable amount of strength, like you're hugging a loved one, but don't "pull" in any particular direction. Imagine you are creating a full boundary of tension around the outside of the body, gently holding the outer edges inward.

In the case of West Stretch, we may stretch the hamstrings somewhat, and the back and the feet and the ankles, and the back, but we aren't necessarily trying to pull them into a longer position. We're just holding a boundary of tension. Inside that boundary, take full, mindful breaths. If you begin to sink farther into the position, that's great. Just let the breath in one at a time.

BREATHING

Allow the inhales to be slow and expansive. Feel your body gently growing outward into the boundaries of its own embrace.

As you exhale, release excess tension from your body in whatever way feels right for you.

Scan your body in the position and "watch" the movement of the breath. See what tension and sensation it encounters; your posterior chain is long, complex, and personal. Intense West Stretch can provide a lot of insight into your own body and tension patterns, if that's what you're after.

OPTIONS

- ◆ If you can't reach your feet, wrap a strap around them. No problem.
- ◆ If sitting on a block was necessary in Staff Pose, stay there for West Stretch, as it may help you locate the "pivot point" of the posture around your pelvis instead of your lower back.

- You can explore making this a completely relaxed position, letting your arms drop to the side and surrendering to gravity. This is often called "Caterpillar" in Yin Yoga, and it serves essentially the same function as Intense West Stretch, just without the muscular engagement.

GOALS

- mindfully and evenly open the posterior chain
- release AO joint tension, in conjunction with full posterior chain release
- establish back-body breathing

Butterfly

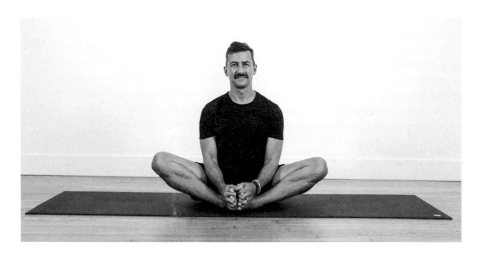

SETUP

From Intense West Stretch, sit up and bend your knees out to the side and put your feet together. With your hands, set a grip across your toes and the pinkie-edges of your feet.

ENTRANCE

Sit tall and roll your shoulders back. As much as is available, set Healthy Neutral in your spine, especially in the position of your skull.

Let your knees fall wide. Don't "push" or anything, just let them move to a position that feels naturally available to you.

BREATHING

The same as in Staff, do some Core Support Breathing. Make this set a little less intense than in Staff. Just encourage the idea of "lift" with both sides of the breath. Think about a jellyfish swimming upward through crystalline blue Caribbean water. With sunbeams. That's you. You're the jellyfish; inhale flap outward to swim upward, exhale flap inward to swim upward. You go get 'em, jelly. You get 'em.

OPTIONS

I love to interlace my fingers between my toes in Butterfly, and highly recommend it. This grip helps open the feet and toes. Your fingers act like those toe-spreaders things from the internet, except they're already attached to your arms, so shipping is free.

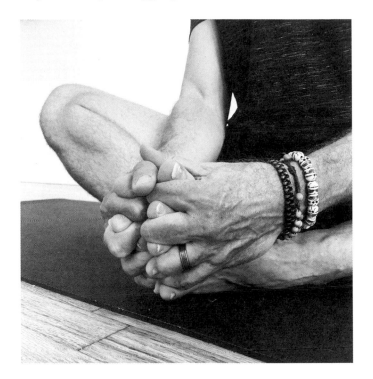

GOALS

- open the adductors
- develop strength in the back in an upright position
- optional toe-spreading
- pattern breathing in Healthy Neutral

Head to Knee

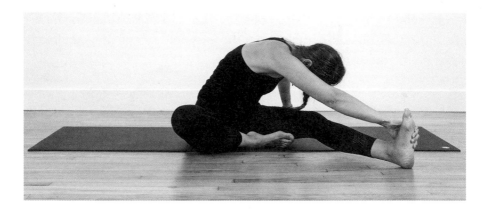

SETUP

From Butterfly, extend your right leg out straight. Put your left foot on your inner right thigh, or wherever it can comfortably rest. (If this doesn't work for your knees, just put both legs straight with your feet wide apart.)

Put your right hand to the right of your hips, maybe a foot away from your body. With your left hand, reach to hold your right foot. (If you can't reach, just reach to your right knee or shin or wherever works for you.)

ENTRANCE

Inhale: Lift your chest and turn your heart toward your right foot.
Exhale: Draw your belly in and gently let your head fall toward your right knee.

ASSESSMENT

Let your left elbow bend down toward the floor, rounding the left shoulder around the rib cage and opening the left side of the upper back.

Don't chase the stretch in your right leg. It will probably happen, and that's fine, but no need to push or pull or anything. Just breathe.

Like in West Stretch, simply give the posture a hug. Create your boundary of tension without pushing the posture in any particular direction.

HUMAN ASYMMETRY

Human beings are, externally, pretty symmetrical organisms. For most of us, our right and left sides are largely identical. Internally, however, it's a different story. Your heart is justified to the left side of your chest. Your liver is larger on the right. Your lungs and diaphragm are organized accordingly, to accommodate these left-right differences. This asymmetry changes the pressure differential in the torso, which changes the way we breathe, which changes all the other stuff too.

In an environment where we move around all day in various directions, these shifts in breathing patterns have negligible effect on our overall tension patterns. However, in sedentary modern life, the shape of the breath takes on a disproportionate influence over your tension patterns. In the absence of constant and variable full-body movement, the little stuff really adds up. This breathing asymmetry can lead to maladaptations, like an uneven back-forth tilt or side-to-side spin of the pelvis.[126]

This is just one way that the tension patterns of the human body can become asymmetrical. As you work with your postures, investigate your own asymmetries. Be patient; they are rarely as simple as "My right leg is stronger than my left." Odds are, if you've got a weak left leg, you have a weak left hip too. Which travels to the shoulders and neck and so on.

We aren't going to tackle asymmetry much in this book—you have seen by now how deeply we can go just focusing Healthy Neutral in the torso—but every now and then you might assess the basics: When you stand or sit upright, are your heart center and pelvis pointed the same way? Do you tend to shift your weight over to one side while waiting in line at Costco?

---

[126] For more information on this phenomenon, I highly recommend reading up on the Pelvic Restoration Institute (www.posturalrestoration.com). They are sort of the leaders in this field, and I think their ideas are pretty genius. I also recommend tracking down a PT who is trained in their method and taking them to the longest coffee date and brain-picking session your schedule will allow.

Which side?[127] Does one shoulder hang lower than the other? Does one shoulder sit farther back than the other, relative to the heart? No need for judgment; we're human, this is simply a helpful process for understanding the conditions of your own body.

---

[127] Betting it's the right.

BREATHING

Easy peasy.

OPTIONS

You can sit on a block for this one, if it helps you lean forward over your leg instead of slouching back. A strap can also be helpful: wrap it around your right foot and hold it in your left hand.

GOALS

- ◆ open the right hamstrings and left adductors
- ◆ open the muscles of the back inside a rotated side bend (particularly the line from the left shoulder to the right hip)

Supine Twist

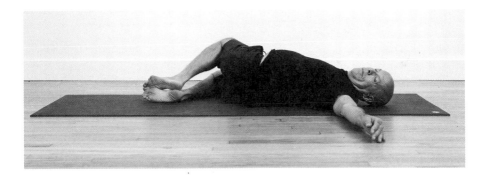

SETUP

Lie down in a comfortable position. Bend your knees and place your feet to the mat close to your hips. Shift your hips to the left edge of the mat and take your arms wide out to the sides.

ENTRANCE

Let your knees fall to the right and turn your chin to the left.

BREATHING

Is great, isn't it? Also, gravity and time.

If you want to prescribe a motion to the breath, think about sending it to the left side of your lower back as well as the left chest.

OPTIONS

Don't think about it too much; you're done. If you have versions of the twist that you really dig (Eagle Legs, Tibetan Weaponry,[128] etc.), go for it.

---

[128] Best yoga pose name of all time, and you will never change my mind. If I ever start a metal glam band, I am naming it Tibetan Weaponry, and we will play songs exclusively about smashing oppressive dictatorships.

GOALS

- ◆ open the top of the chest on the left side
- ◆ open the side bodies and lower back
- ◆ relax the whole system

GRAVITY, BREATHING, AND TIME

In our world of individualism and achievement and work ethic and "crushing life" and whatever, we might get the idea that the most influential thing in our life is inside our skull. And that's not totally wrong. Choices matter, responsibility matters, beliefs matter. And our brain—or our mind, really, because they're not the same thing—is indeed super important. In terms of the story of our life, the narrative of identity, the choices we make are primary.

But there is much more going on than our story. Our identity narratives are only part of the picture. Behind the world of the conscious day-to-day grind, a whole world of influence and interaction is rolling on. For example, the weight of your body—its attraction to the earth—is keeping it healthy. Pressure heals your bones, and the resistance of gravity trains your muscles. Astronauts, for example, can lose muscle mass and even develop vision problems after a long time in space, because the muscles that move and focus the human eye are designed to work in relation to gravity.

We might consider that some of the things that really change us are unconscious or beyond our capacity to change. Gravity changes us. Breathing changes us. Time changes us. Only breathing can be intentionally modified while on earth, and even then, you wouldn't want to live your whole life in a state of constant breath control.

By inviting the profound power of these elements into our practice, engaging their perpetual influence on us directly, we acknowledge a simple reality about our daily lives. Much of what determines the quality of our existence as human beings happens outside the boundaries of our mental narratives of identity and control.

Corpse

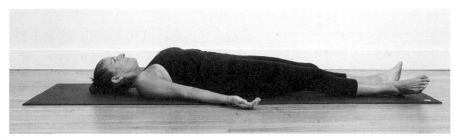

Play dead.

> *Life is not a puzzle; it's a mystery.*
>
> —RABBI DAVID WOLPE

There is an important Rule of Three that I've been avoiding up until now, and it has to do with how and why we put together patterns.

A lot of what we've tried to do together in this book is investigate patterns in human bodies, minds, and behaviors. Patterns are both real and not. They are in some ways the creation of the human mind: our brains use patterns to form our perception of the world, create meaning, and predict the future. If you push a Volvo off a fjord, you know it will fall into the ocean below, because in the past gravity has been consistent. Without support, things move downward at a very predictable rate. You know this because of a pattern of experience. Without this pattern and others like it, you and I would have no concept of the rules of reality.

Yoga can be a method of reforming patterns. Change your physical behavior, and you change your body patterns. Change what you read, whose twitter feed you follow, what news channel you watch, or how often you meditate, and you'll change the patterns of your mind. We can use patterns to interpret reality, to figure out the world around us. In an infinite field of information, we gird our psyches from overload by organizing patterns from sensory input. This is how we form concepts like oceans, waves, tides, beaches, and sunsets. It is how we analyze the weather. Pattern formation is the basis of each and every one of our human relationships.

But it is important to acknowledge our limitations. Patterns are not perfect. Since the patterns of our experience are built by and for our limited minds, they cannot fully integrate the complexity of reality. Chaos is central to the system, and we should be glad for it. If patterns or logic or data analysis could be truly predictive—if there were no chaos—we would live in a world without freedom or choice.

Life is not a puzzle; it is a mystery. We will never put the whole picture together. We do our best within the unknown, holding out candles within an infinite cave, but we should not deceive ourselves: the darkness will remain, largely, a mystery. We will never know eternity.

And so it goes on. A teacher of mine used to say, "It's about radical faith, and radical doubt." You know, and then you don't. You know. And then you don't. Back and forth, up and down. The vibration, *spanda,* doesn't stop. So, as it keeps going, we keep going. When you feel like you know something, go looking for the mystery. When you feel like you're in the mystery, go looking for the pattern. In a way, this may be the inhale and exhale of the philosophical life. Catch and release. Climb and fall. Wake and sleep. When you recall your dreams, what is most interesting to you? What fades away?

As we practice, I invite you to explore what patterns, ideas, and perspectives resonate with you. What map of reality meets your felt experience of it? There is no absolute answer, only the process of engagement. We are creatures of knowledge and ignorance at once. Hold fast and be moved, balance experimentation with tradition, balance discipline with curiosity, keep what works for you and let what does not recede. And perhaps maintain an understanding that we will never be finished, only changed into something new, and upon this new thing we will build the next change.

The work, in this light, is to participate, investigate, and choose our manner of being as best we can, knowing that we must limit our access to the infinite in each moment; that being human means creating shapes from the shapeless, signs out of dust, gods out of chaos, and carrying on regardless.

Take your time. And as you choose to go, go in peace.

A THEORY OF RELATIVITY IN THE TIME OF EXPONENTIAL GROWTH

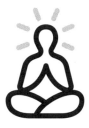

THE STORIES MONKEYS TELL

L et's imagine you're a monkey. And it's great: you live in the trees and cavort with other monkeys, and your prehensile tail is glorious, and everything is just as good as Planet Earth makes it look. One morning you get hungry for mangoes, like monkeys do. But there are hawks that live near the mango trees. And these hawks eat monkeys, which is lame and painful and also quite fatal, so you want nothing to do with them. In this case, you would do well to have some ideas in your monkey brain about what hawks are and how to avoid them.

So, OK, let's say you and your monkey friends notice there's a *swoosh* sound whenever a hawk is nearby. Since you're a monkey, you don't really understand sound waves or the semifluid dynamics of air. But you do have the basic information that hawks and *swoosh* sounds arrive at the same time. So you might look up and run your cute little black monkey fingers through your silver chin-hairs and, in your monkey wisdom, come up with a story that says *Hawks are made out of swoosh sounds.* This story would be wrong, of course.[129] However, it would contain the basic information you need to survive, which is *Swoosh sounds mean a hawk is nearby.*

For monkeys, surviving the jungle is far more important than comprehending it, so if your story has the necessary survival information, it

---

[129] Hawks are most likely made out of lightning, gumption, and zip ties.

doesn't need to be "right." It just needs to help you survive. And then you can teach your monkey kids this story about hawks, and maybe over time the story becomes part of the greater monkey culture. This is one way an illusion can become a mainstream idea: the illusion is useful enough to survive, replicate, and prosper.

But what happens when a hawk goes flying over the mango tree and suddenly gets a brain aneurysm and—*swoosh*—it falls to the ground, and for the first time in your glorious monkey life, you get to see an honest-to-gracious hawk up close and personal? Which is cool, but also maybe a little confusing because it's right there in front of you in the dirt, and you don't hear any *swoosh*. That's odd, you think. After all, aren't hawks made out of *swoosh*?

Confronted with this new information, what do you do with your story about hawks? If we were purely rational monkeys, we would immediately revise our hawk story. Maybe we'd say, "Oh … OK. We had the hawk thing wrong. Turns out hawks weren't made of *swoosh* at all. Gotta be made out of something else entirely. Can someone call Loretta and tell her we need to change the stories about hawks? Yeah, scrap the *swoosh* thing. No *swoosh*. It looks like this hawk is a bat that is covered in tiny ferns … that's the new story. Hawks are bats covered in tiny ferns, best we can tell."

That sort of response would be, in a way, how humans have done science throughout history. Have a wrong idea, get new evidence, revise your old wrong idea into a better idea that is *also wrong* but closer to reality. And if you do this a whole lot of times, through progressively less-wrong ideas, you may eventually land on the right answer. A hawk is not a bat covered in ferns; a hawk is a bird. But "bat covered in ferns" is a more accurate description of a hawk than "swoosh."[130]

---

[130] I can hear some objections to this sentence, already. There might be a philosopher or guru out there who wants to make the point that *birds only exist in the present moment, and there is no non-arbitrary distinction between a being in the world and the sound it creates in the present moment, so when a hawk makes a* swoosh *it is legitimate to say the hawk and the* swoosh *are one and the same!* This might be a compelling idea to unpack, theoretically. And though it's a fun way to explore our experience of the world, it's not actually that helpful in understanding the hawk. (Lots of things go *swoosh* in the air.)

But we might not do science. Science is just one way of thinking. We might come up with a new twist on the old story, just to protect the illusion. We might say something like, "OK, fellow monkeys. We all know hawks are definitely made of *swoosh*. There's no question there. So why is there no swooshing now? New idea: when hawks die the ground mixes with the *swoosh* and turns it into *thud*. This hawk is made out of *thud* now. Don't touch it or you'll be infected and make *thud* everywhere you go because the *thud* is contagious."

What started out as a simple explanation for the hawk-*swoosh* association is now complicated. And the more we learn about hawks, the more complex our story will become. More and more magical onomatopoeias will become necessary to maintain our first little story that hawks are made of *swoosh*.

Luckily, as far as we can tell, monkeys don't actually do this. Unluckily, human beings very much do. We create all kinds of stories about the world and our place in it. We conjure narratives about things like who we are, what we believe, what a person is, what a community is, where we are going, and where we have been. Some of these stories are chosen; some are given. Some are faithful to reality, and some are not.

Yoga teaches us that we can assess our stories and reform our ideas about the world. Maya, the illusion that dances before us all, is intoxicating but not entirely insurmountable. Should we look, and allow our patterns of thought and perception to evolve, we may discover new and vital realities about ourselves and our world. There's always something to find, because every pattern of awareness has a blind spot.

But it's hard. Much of the work of self-discovery and illusion is embarrassing. Human beings are complicated things. We are very good at constructing stories that protect our existing ideas, reinforce our belief systems, and deny contrary evidence. The mind is tricky this way. People who practice mindfulness understand that the chattering monkey inside the human skull is less concerned with truth than it is with self-defense. It does not want to look for blind spots; it wants to survive.

But truth matters. The capacity to honestly and humbly explore experience, to repattern ourselves and grow closer to reality, is profound. And to do so intentionally is, as far as we can tell, a distinctly human trait. We can choose to repattern. It's usually harder than we like to admit—sometimes it takes a major wake-up call like an injury or a social shift—but it can be done. The work of yoga, meditation, mindfulness, therapy, and self-help all operate on this principle; we can learn more honest, compassionate, comprehensive ways of engaging our experience in the great interconnected space of this reality.

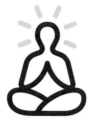

WITHIN THE GREAT JOSEPHINE

S o far, we have discussed patterns primarily in terms of three-dimensional shapes: your body patterns are three-dimensional shapes, yoga poses are three-dimensional shapes, and the grooves in your brain are three-dimensional shapes. (We don't really know if thoughts have three-dimensional shapes, but they—at the very least—correlate with three-dimensional shapes in your gray matter. Beyond that threshold we are jettisoned into the realm of the speculative, the metaphysical, and the weird.)

But we have also touched a few times on how patterns move in the fourth dimension: time. Habits and rituals are patterns of action, written on the canvas of time. And just like their 3-D brethren, the various elements of 4-D patterns are both connected and distinct. They influence each other because they are deeply interwoven. The past begets the present, the present creates the future. The future calls the present forward (what are your dreams, my friend?) and the present defines the past.

Time, see, is a sort of Josephine. The present and past and future are all components of a larger whole. We pull this Josephine apart and inspect individual moments because that's all our brains can handle, but if you push on one part of eternity, the rest of it will bend.

Let me ask you this: when does an event begin? When you go to the grocery store, when does the "trip to the grocery store" start? When you make a list? When you choose to leave? When you get on your bike? When you walk through the doors? When you select your first item?

How long does one moment last? What is the duration of "the present"?[131]

The Law of Karma says that what we do with our small, seemingly insignificant moment in this eternal process matters. Human beings are capable of shaping the world through choice: how we choose to act, what patterns of behavior we engage, etc. These things have real and lasting effects because they touch all of time. Everything inside of "now" comes from everything before and goes on forever.

On a genetic level, a wonderful game is at play here. The past determines what genetic code arrives in the present moment; the present—through both natural selection and gene expression[132]—manifests and transmits those genes; the future blooms from this transmission. Evolution, in this sense, is a pattern in the fourth dimension. Before life sprung up in the primordial muck and biological evolution began, chemical reactions were whirring in the black waters and the brilliant stars, and physics—quantum and mechanical both—was shaping the cosmos. The game of connection and influence ripples throughout the patterns of time and will continue ad infinitum.

Consider for a moment, if you will, that what you do today—right now—will reverberate forever. This breath? It contains the entirety of the past, and it will carry on forever. Even when it ceases to be oxygen and carbon dioxide, even when the earth itself is gone, this exhale right here will influence the great, ongoing Josephine. If we honestly engage this idea, what does it mean about who we are and how we live? What does it mean about the choices we make?

---

[131] I swear to God I'm not high right now. I don't get high. No judgment at all about it, it's just me. It makes me paranoid. I get quiet and hungry and secretly suspect everyone else in the room is plotting some kind of "failed person" ceremony about me. Or they're already having it in their minds. Or whenever I go to the bathroom they snicker and point. Which, I get, is shamefully self-centered and ma-a-aybe says something about me as an individual? Like, I don't know, maybe there's some personal stuff I should be working on? Anyways, if you want to know what my brain is like when I'm high, reread this footnote twelve times and then eat a whole jar of queso with a spoon.

[132] Recommendation: Go down a rabbit hole on "gene expression" if you have not already. It's amazing.

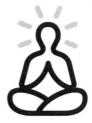

HEAT IN THE TIME OF HEAT

took my first hot yoga class on December 26, 2010. I had developed terrible shin splints from a failed attempt at obsessive running (bad movement patterns at the time, it turns out) and my brother dragged me to a Bikram Yoga studio in the heart of Philadelphia. I sweat buckets, hated life, crashed in a puddle, and fell in love with the whole thing. Within a year I was a certified Bikram Yoga instructor. Six months later I opened a studio, with that very same brother.

I have a deep appreciation for the heat. It has certainly helped shape who I am today. In many ways, it opened my heart. It undeniably makes you more limber and promotes sweat (which is good).[133] And your body's capillary response to extreme heat[134] increases blood flow to the muscles, so soft tissue heals more effectively when exposed to heat.

I spent many years preaching the Gospel of Heat, even after I left the Bikram Yoga world and developed the Foundations of Repatterning. But a funny thing happened to me a little while ago; I saw through an illusion of mine. I was forced to confront my own hypocrisy, with much embarrassment.

---

[133] Stay hydrated, my friends.

[134] Vasodilation, during which the capillaries expand and allow more blood to flow to the surface of the skin, which helps move heat out from the core of the body to its exterior, and then out into the environment through the skin.

During the spring and summer of 2020—while writing this book—I had to shut down my hot yoga studio because, as you may have heard, there was a global pandemic. I learned all kinds of things during that time, like what it's like to teach Foundations to a webcam (not awesome) and how a yoga room starts to feel a little haunted after a month or so without students. I also learned we could, as a studio family, discover just as much value from outdoor classes as we did in the hot room.

And then, as I learned how much an energy bill craters when you don't create extreme artificial heat, I witnessed the terrible consequences of science denial in real time. (In case my sarcasm and unearned confidence haven't cued you in yet, I'm from the United States.[135]) In the great pause of the pandemic, as hundreds of thousands of Americans died because people didn't want to acknowledge the inconvenient prevalence of a deadly virus, I was given a view to one of my personal failures. I too had avoided inconvenient truths. Realities that, when fully integrated, demanded I change the way I live. A human being can only deny the truth for so long.

One of the 4-D patterns of life is that, after it ends, organic matter that is not consumed by other life decays and transmutes into other forms. On a long enough time horizon, some of this organic matter is buried by sediment and turns into crude oil. One of the patterns of modern civilization is to extract this oil from underground and burn it for energy.

long rhetorical pause
thousand-yard stare
slow inhale

There is currently no question that human fossil fuel usage is changing the climate, and that those changes will have disastrous effects on our global Josephine, the biosphere. A vital effort to reduce emissions is ongoing and essential to the well-being of living things across the planet.

---

[135] Also I'm a cis white male so, like, I'm writing you this postcard from atop Mount Privilege where, in case you're wondering, the only potable water comes from the Well of Impending Doom.

Human beings with less access to resources—those who are least responsible for this calamity—are at special risk of famine, drought, displacement, and death. We[136] affect their long-term well-being with our actions. To needlessly consume energy is to perform harm on people who quite literally cannot defend themselves.

long rhetorical pause
taking the temperature of the room, now[137]

If this feels like a wild left-turn in your yoga book; I get it. If your neck is sore from the whiplash, I understand. After all, we were having such a good time, weren't we?[138] What's with the politics? What does this have to do with repatterning and Healthy Neutral and, you know … lunges?

Tapestry

So far, we've had a bunch of conversations about how context changes us. Our world shapes us both mentally and physically. Modernity has placed particular and unique strains on our human bodies and minds, and we have had to adjust accordingly. Some of these adjustments have been tough on us. We weren't made to eat processed food or live in boxes or stare at screens for hours each day. And yet, here we are.

Our context is not simply modernity or civilization, though. It is far larger than that. It encompasses all phenomena—biological, chemical, and physical—on this remarkable blue marble. (Plus, very importantly, the sun.[139]) Every organism on the planet has been influenced somehow

---

[136] I.e. yoga students pretty much anywhere in the Western world, no matter where you land on the economic spectrum. If you have the means and time to pay for yoga, you are pretty much super-wealthy in the global sense and have a disproportionate influence on things like climate change and environmental politics.

[137] Unintentional puns are the best puns.

[138] *Weren't we?*

[139] If you want to get really out there, we could say the whole universe is involved. Because it is. But let's keep this part manageable, yeah?

by the advancement of civilization. Every plant and animal, every bacteria and fungus the world over is part of this changing world. Some changes lead to growth; jellyfish have adapted to warmer ocean waters and are flourishing now more than any other time in their known history. Sometimes these changes lead to death; as the ice caps melt, polar bears can't evolve fast enough to account for the loss of their wintry habitat and natural prey. You've seen the pictures.

Or, to keep on brand: If there is such a thing as Healthy Neutral in the natural world, we are moving away from it at high speeds.

We are woven into the biosphere in both time and space. A human being is an individual and a component. You are your own thing, and you are also part of something much greater than any single human being. You are, now and always, both. If through our practice we witness the interconnected nature of our bodies and actions, we might begin to see other parts of our existence similarly. The trees breathe out what we breathe in. The cattle change the soil, which changes the plants, which changes the food, which changes the cattle. The yoga heating unit changes the energy demand, which changes the power plant, which changes the air quality, which changes the yoga. We pay for yoga with money that is regulated by the government. We (usually) heat our hot yoga studios with carbon.

It's likely that at least one molecule of the Buddha's first exhale after attaining enlightenment is in your lungs right now.[140] There is no extricating ourselves from … well … whatever this all is.

> The loom—tantra—weaves us into the tapestry of reality. Our actions—karma—have consequences. The idea that we are fundamentally separate from all things is an illusion—maya.

We cannot return to an ancient form of life, nor escape the digital age, nor transcend the political and social challenges of our time. We must engage things as they are, from where we are. Politics and environment and nature and yoga—they're all part of the life we live today. You can't

---

[140] James Lloyd, "Are We Really Breathing Caesar's Last Breath?" *Science Focus* 310 (2017), https://tinyurl.com/y66uvxzd.

actually pull this Josephine apart, friend. It's all one thing. Politics and environment and yoga practice are all part of the same comprehensive whole. You can't really build walls around them, only illusions, because they're not separate things. I've heard many people express a desire to keep politics out of yoga, as the base and mundane may have some kind of corruptive influence on the sacred. But yoga *is* politics, if only because yoga is part of the world. If you ask me,[141] a yoga practice that pretends to exist independent of our context is not a path out of illusion, but a path into its depths.[142]

I ignored the impact of hot yoga on the biosphere because I wanted my work to be separate from the turning of the world. My desires birthed illusion, and I lived within that illusion for many years. The hawks were made of *swoosh*. So it goes; I am a human being.

But once you let the truth in, it changes you.

---

[141] Which, I'm sure you've realized by now, is a highly questionable move…

[142] If this all sounds preachy, please keep in mind that I knew about climate change for many years before owning the implications of the truth. I have zero moral high ground here; the only way I ever really learn anything is by messing up. Better late than never.

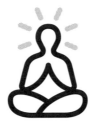

PRAXIS

For many years I practiced a yoga that was almost exclusively about me. And that wasn't all bad. I needed to learn self-care. But if we walk down this road for long enough, it turns. We see ourselves from different horizons. Sometimes the going gets hard and we may get tempted to turn back. We often avoid the things that will truly change us, because they are real and scary. Or because they're inconvenient. Or just because changing ourselves means giving up something we really, really, really like. Like new spandex or meat or extreme artificial heat.

And you don't have to give everything up. Yoga works wherever you apply yourself to it with intelligence and care. For sure, we workshopped and cultivated the Foundations practice in hot yoga studios. It was born in the furnace, but it does not necessarily need to stay there. It's just fine wherever. None of the poses in this practice require extreme temperatures in order to be functional or safe.[143] You don't have to get sweat in your eyes to see the truth.

I'm not saying you have to stop practicing hot yoga. However, if we are truly committed to a powerful practice, if we are willing to let our explorations repattern the way we act and think in the world, if we are capable of seeing how essentially we are connected, and if we can honestly assess our relationship to context, according to the challenges of the present day, I think it becomes pretty difficult to morally justify a hot yoga ritual.

This is only one example of the way a yoga practice, as an investigation into the nature of life, can inform our moral and political existence. The fundamental questions remain in any context. When we interrogate our illusions and our desires, what do we find? What can we change? What must we do? This kind of practice will pervade and reform our approach to the challenges of our own time. Be it racism or homophobia or sea turtles or wealth distribution or whether or not to use the fire hoses on indigenous people protesting the theft and desecration of their land, we may find clarity in all of it through an honest practice.

I want to be clear on something. I'm not saying that solving climate change is solely the responsibility of individual people. The real issue is endemic to our economic structure and isn't simply a "personal choice" issue. To actually save our biosphere from collapse, we will have to revolutionize the way global power systems function and sustain themselves. Stopping a hot yoga practice ain't the answer. But real change will require a shift in mind-set, a unified global embrace of the challenges of our time.

---

[143] For the record: I have never encountered a yoga pose that is fundamentally safe in a hot room and unsafe in a not-hot room. That's ... not a thing. Warming up before you perform any athletic activity is usually helpful but not required. You can run down the block without warming up; you can climb a tree without warming up; etc. Warming the body helps, but there's no reason to forbid activities without it. Same with yoga poses. You don't *have* to be warm to avoid hurting yourself. In fact, if you're not all toasty and limber, you might have to slow down and pay more attention to *Oh, no, now you're moving slowly and paying attention to your feelings.* And besides, there are lots of ways to heat the body that don't involve artificial heat (see: *Salutations, Sun*).

Becoming part of the tapestry of change is a personal choice. Climate solutions will require that we investigate how we think about social and ecological responsibility on a broad scale. Basically, we must change our culture. And one of the things we must change is our collective desire to prioritize comfort and convenience.

Yoga brings us closer to real experience, away from the illusions we conjure to preserve our own routines, preferences, and habits. And the thing about getting closer to experience is, as far as I can tell, it doesn't provide many clean answers. In fact, it often just makes the questions more pressing: Do I like hot yoga more than not-hot yoga? You're goddamn right I do. Do I want to sweat seven pounds of water weight and collapse in a demented heap at the end of a hard day? Nothing sounds better. Does my hot yoga practice make me happier or even more calm? Can't deny it. But do these benefits override the broader concerns? Global concerns? Concerns for the future of life on this planet? What does my love for sweaty bliss mean in a world where energy expenditure is already causing species extinction, famine, and refugee crises? When we choose to be honest and humble in the face of life, as it is, we often find ourselves challenged to become agents of a new way of being.

I'm telling you this because my best teachers were the ones who spoke their truths out loud. They were gentle when they needed to be gentle and firm when they needed to be firm. They chose compassion over comfort and honesty over good vibes every time. I am inspired by them to speak my own part.

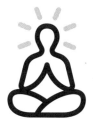

ON PATIENCE, JOY,
AND ENDINGS

When we dive into the practice of repatterning, the first thing we learn is how hard it is. To challenge our habits and confront our limitations is arduous work, and sort of contrary to the impulses of our lizard-brains. Lizards are creatures of habit and, on a lizard level, so are we all. But this work doesn't have to be filled with suffering or agony. It can be fun. If we can change our minds about the meaning of stretching pain, we can change our minds about discipline, routine, and the value of slow transformation.

Little victories operate like hedge funds.[144] They leverage compounding interest. A 2 percent change every few months might seem small now, but over time it creates remarkable growth. The main thing is to stay with it as best you can. There are a lot of details and annoying corrections in the posture section of this book.[145] You get to work on them as you like, over time. Choose what suits you and your body. Assess yourself

---

[144] Hail Satan!

[145] One reader was all, like, "Bro. You are seriously overteaching these postures." And I was, like, "I know; isn't it great?" Because, you know, communication skills.

regularly, with a kind eye. You're already perfect, and you have room for improvement. Just like everyone.

If working with your patterns gets challenging, reach out for assistance. There are loads of amazing teachers out there. If you find someone who helps you see the good in you, consider them wise. Also, from time to time, take a breather. Have a banana. Remember, you're a human being, and human beings are awesome. We are statistical miracles within unfathomable space. Keep in mind that an explosion in the middle of nothingness brought forth not only hydrogen atoms but eyeballs and kneecaps. That you're here at all makes no goddamn sense, which is why it's so goddamn cool.

So, make sure there is some joy in your practice. Take it seriously, and then don't. Follow the Rule of Three. Some days maybe you put on Gregorian chant as your yoga music. Some days maybe it's Kelly Clarkson. (I won't tell you which of these represents joy and which represents seriousness; you do you.) Some days, do the poses with your most intense discipline. Some days just let it move through you. Some days cry. Some days smile. Other days smile and cry at the same time and maybe take a second to marvel at how ridiculous and strange it is to be embodied at all.

And don't forget that one day, after all the mindfulness and the back bends and the kale smoothies, you won't be embodied anymore. You will melt back into the whole thing, and the dissolution of your personal patterns will ripple and shape and inform all the rest, forever. Which is good and bad. Hard and easy. Here and gone.

How Do Things End?

So. That's it. That's the book. Time to wrap things up and go climb a tree, I guess. If you've made it to the end with me, I'm truly honored. What you do matters, and I'm humbled that you've done whatever this is with me for this long.

Should we ever find one another out there in the tangle of automobiles and Wi-Fi and birds, I hope we can share the practice. Or maybe just a terrible joke. That would be pretty great.

We're already sharing the whole world.

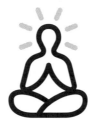

EPILOGUE

Down the hill to the waterfront and across the blue-white lake, beneath the hovering ghost of morning fog, through the softwood regrowth that hangs at angles from the cracks in the shale, over the highway and past the single traffic light marking a pale yellow pulse in the heart of Elizabethtown, up around the bend on the logging road, you'll find a trail. Take it. It's well marked and boot-worn; the going will be fair enough.

Three miles back in the forest and up the mountain more than a thousand feet, the wind is gone and the air smells like other seasons. Wet moss and the decay of leaves, spring and autumn both. Find the stream with the makeshift log bridge. There, step off the trail and follow the water uphill a ways, maybe a hundred yards. Maybe more, if you like.

Search the stream for a large stone, manageable with good weight. It will be there. Lift it from the cold water, see the mud unbind and billow and disperse like smoke to the wind. Do not despair the stoneflies.

Carry this secret upstream, perhaps ten paces. Find a spot where the sounds are just right and with great ceremony—or none at all—return it to the water. It is embraced by the current now, folded again into the way of things, both obstacle and terrain. If you are the sort, you might say a prayer. Some choose to sing.

Nothing and everything has happened. You have done an insignificant thing, performed a trifle, come all this way for no good reason. So stay and watch. Watch the stream as it ripples around the stone, assumes an original turbulence, and discovers a new route toward its imperative. Water flows downhill. Remember now that the combination of water and time has shaped the planet, carved Champlain and the Grand Canyon both. The stream will wear away the boundaries of rock and soil alike and make new edges below, new fault lines and sedimentary deposits, new corners for the crawdads, new riptides for pollen and foam.

Perhaps just now you have divided the future, turned a key in the ecosystem, and this simple, insignificant act will prove the tipping point in next spring's floods. Maybe someday, miles from here, the stream will split in two. A child will spring from this mother. The white-tailed deer will drink from virgin brooks and the mayflies will swarm them within unfamiliar clearings. Burrows will be inundated, a field of flowers drowned. New forms will appear and dissolve into the next as generations, evolution in the family of all things. This will carry on for earth's eternity.

Part of this eternity will be today. Part of it will be you. You will never know for sure which part.

APPENDIX
THE FOUNDATIONS OF REPATTERNING: SEQUENCE OPTIONS

Key

* Poses listed with a dash mean the postures "flow" into one another without stopping to reset.

* (R) means do the right side of a pose; (L) means do the left side.

* (R-L) means when you're done on one side of a pose or set, reset and then go back and do the other side.

* (S) means take a brief rest in either Savasana or lying prone between poses.

* (2) means do two sets of the pose.

* Take a short break, just a breath or two, between each step in the sequence.

75–90 Minutes

This is the standard version for Foundations of Repatterning. It provides the most benefit, so if you really want to get down to business, this is the sequence for you. You can make it longer or shorter depending on how long you choose to hold the poses, how long you allow yourself to reset between postures, and if you choose to integrate a brief sitting period (kneeling meditation) toward the end of the class.

Between each set, pause a moment and take a breath.

- Pulling Down the Heavens (3)
- Reverse Anatomical Breathing (7–12)
- side bends—back bend—forward fold (2)
- Chair—Chair on Toes—Power Pose—Revolved Lunge (R-L)
- Eagle (R-L, 2)
- Big Toe Pose (R-L)
- Revolved Big Toe Pose (R-L)
- Core Strength Quad Stretch—Standing Bow (R-L, 2)
- Airplane—Revolved Half Moon (R-L, 2)
- Three-Legged Dog—Vitruvian Person—mid-stance fold
- Warrior 2—Warrior Triangle (R-L, 2)
- Pyramid—Revolved Triangle (R-L, 2)
- Tree (R-L)
- Corpse (2 minutes)
- Wind Removing (R-L)
- Wind Removing (both legs)
- Bridge (2)
- Plunge (S)
- Cobra (2, S)
- Crocodile (2, S)
- Bow (2, S)
- Child
- Forearm Plank—Dolphin
- Child
- Dog—Pigeon (R-L)
- Supine Warrior
- Half Tortoise
- Camel
- Wild Child (or Screaming Child)
- optional: kneeling meditation (1–5 minutes)
- Staff
- Intense West Stretch
- Butterfly (R-L)
- Head to Knee (R-L, S)
- Supine Twist (R-L)
- Corpse

60 Minutes

This is a version of the 75–90 Minutes class where everything is condensed into one set. In a couple of cases, poses have been combined, but for the most part it's very similar.

- Pulling Down the Heavens (3)
- Reverse Anatomical Breathing (7)
- side bends—back bend—forward fold
- Chair—Chair on Toes—Power Pose—Revolved Lunge (R-L)
- Eagle (R-L)
- Big Toe Pose—Revolved Big Toe Pose (R-L)
- Core Strength Quad Stretch—Standing Bow (R-L)
- Airplane—Revolved Half Moon (R-L)
- Three-Legged Dog—Vitruvian Person—mid-stance fold
- Warrior 2—Warrior Triangle (R-L)
- Pyramid—Revolved Triangle (R-L)
- Tree (R-L)
- Corpse (2 minutes)
- Wind Removing (R-L)
- Wind Removing (both legs)
- Bridge
- Plunge
- Cobra (S)
- Crocodile (S)
- Bow (S)
- Child
- Forearm Plank—Dolphin
- Child
- Dog—Pigeon (R-L)
- Supine Warrior
- Half Tortoise
- Camel
- Wild Child (or Screaming Child)
- Staff
- Intense West Stretch
- Butterfly (R-L)
- Head to Knee (R-L, S)
- Supine Twist (R-L)
- Corpse

30 Minutes

We get this into 30 minutes by keeping it moving, never holding any pose too long, and making smooth transitions. A few sequencing elements are modified to make things work together, especially in the separate-leg work.

- Pulling Down the Heavens
- Reverse Anatomical Breathing
- side bends—back bend—forward fold—Chair—Chair on Toes—Power Pose—Revolved Lunge—Eagle (R-L)
- Big Toe Pose—Revolved Big Toe Pose (R-L)
- Core Strength Quad Stretch—Standing Bow—Airplane—Revolved Half Moon (R-L)
- Three-Legged Dog—Warrior 2 (R)—Warrior Triangle (R)—Warrior 2 (L)—Warrior Triangle (L)—Vitruvian Person—mid-stance fold—Pyramid (R)—Revolved Triangle (R)—Pyramid (L)—Revolved Triangle (L)
- Tree (R-L)
- Cobra

- Crocodile
- Bow
- Child
- Forearm Plank—Dolphin
- Child
- Dog—Pigeon (R-L)
- Supine Warrior
- Half Tortoise
- Camel
- Wild Child (or Screaming Child)
- Staff
- Intense West Stretch
- Wind Removing (R-L)
- Wind Removing (both legs)
- Plunge
- Bridge
- Supine Twist (R-L)
- Corpse

BIBLIOGRAPHY

Bowman, Katy. *Move Your DNA: Restore Your Health through Natural Movement.* Carlsborg, WA: Propriometrics Press, 2017.

Contreras, Bret, and Glen Cordoza. *Glute Lab: The Art and Science of Strength and Physique Training.* Las Vegas, NV: Victory Belt, 2019.

Duthon, Victoria B., Caecilia Charbonnier, Frank C. Kolo, Elia Coppens, Pierre Hoffmeyer, and Jacques Menetrey. "Correlation of Clinical and Magnetic Resonance Imaging Findings in Hips of Elite Female Ballet Dancers." *Journal of Arthroscopy and Related Surgery* 29:3 (March 2013), 411–19. doi:10.1016/j.arthro.2012.10.012.

Hedley, Gil. *Fascia and Stretching: The Fuzz Speech.* Video. February 7, 2009. https://youtu.be/_FtSP-tkSug.

Iyengar, B. K. S. *Light on Yoga: Yoga Dipika.* London: Allen & Unwin, 1966.

Klappenbach, Laura. "Understanding Sexual Dimorphism." ThoughtCo. February 19, 2019. https://tinyurl.com/y6o5rwax.

Lephart, Scott M., Cheryl M. Ferris, Bryan L. Riemann, Joseph B. Myers, and Freddie H. Fu. "Gender Differences in Strength and Lower Extremity Kinematics during Landing." *Clinical Orthopaedics and Related Research* 401 (August 2002): 162–69. https://tinyurl.com/y6gwpj6x.

Lloyd, James. "Are We Really Breathing Caesar's Last Breath?" *Science Focus* 310 (2017). https://tinyurl.com/y66uvxzd.

Marshall, Ron. *Marketing Survival in a Digital World.* Springfield, MO: Big RAM, 2013.

McNevin, Nancy H., and Gabriele Wulf. "Attentional Focus on Supra-postural Tasks Affects Postural Control." *Human Movement Science* 21:2 (2002): 187–202. doi:10.1016/S0167-9457(02)00095-7.

Myers, Thomas W. *Anatomy Trains.* London: Primal Pictures, 2004.

Shahar, David, and Mark G. L. Sayers. "Prominent Exostosis Projecting from the Occipital Squama More Substantial and Prevalent in Young Adult Than Older Age Groups." *Scientific Reports* 8:3354 (2018). doi:10.1038/s41598-018-21625-1.

Wallace, David Foster. *Infinite Jest*. New York: Little, Brown, 1996.

ABOUT THE AUTHORS

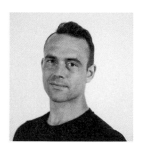 Kyle Ferguson (E-RYT 200) is the creator and director of Second Circle Yoga in Burlington, Vermont. Originally certified in Bikram Yoga in 2011, Kyle received additional teaching certifications in Alignment-Based Hatha Yoga (Maha Yoga, 2015), and Yin Yoga (Yoga Home, 2018). He is a graduate of the University of Pennsylvania's Mindfulness-Based Stress Relief program, and has completed the Zen Mountain Monastery's Introduction to Zen Practice. In 2018, he created Second Circle Yoga in Vermont with the aim of developing a powerful, modern, scientifically informed practice for hot yoga enthusiasts everywhere.

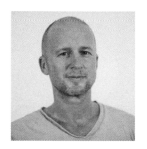 Anthony Grudin is the author of *Warhol's Working Class: Pop Art and Egalitarianism* (University of Chicago Press, 2017) and *Animal Warhol,* forthcoming from the University of California Press in 2022.

About North Atlantic Books

North Atlantic Books (NAB) is an independent, nonprofit publisher committed to a bold exploration of the relationships between mind, body, spirit, and nature. Founded in 1974, NAB aims to nurture a holistic view of the arts, sciences, humanities, and healing. To make a donation or to learn more about our books, authors, events, and newsletter, please visit www.northatlanticbooks.com.

North Atlantic Books is a 501(c)(3) nonprofit educational organization that promotes cross-cultural perspectives linking scientific, social, and artistic fields. To learn how you can support us, please visit our website.